IMPORTANT
INFORMATION

Doctor

Name_____

Address_____

Telephone number_____

Hospital

Emergency room telephone number_____

Police Department

Telephone number_____

Fire Department

Telephone number_____

Neighbor to Be Called in Emergency

Name_____

Address_____

Telephone number_____

Poison Control

Telephone number_____

Also by Jeffrey L. Brown

Telephone Medicine:
A Practical Guide to
Pediatric Telephone Advice

THE COMPLETE PARENTS' GUIDE TO TELEPHONE MEDICINE:
How, When and Why to Call Your Child's Doctor

A Ready Reference for:
Childhood Illnesses
Common Emergencies
Newborn Infant Care
Psychological and Behavior Problems

Jeffrey L. Brown, M.D., F.A.A.P.

A PERIGEE BOOK

Perigee Books
are published by
G. P. Putnam's Sons
200 Madison Avenue
New York, New York 10016

Library of Congress Cataloging in Publication Data

Brown, Jeffrey L.
The complete parents' guide to telephone medicine.

1. Children—Diseases. 2. Pediatric emergencies.
3. Communication in pediatrics. 4. Telephone in medicine.
I. Title.
RJ61.B87   1981   618.92   81-8552
ISBN 0-399-50582-2   AACR2

First Perigee printing, 1982
Printed in the United States of America

Fifth Impression

Dedicated to
my wonderful parents, Joel and Edna;
and to my very understanding family
Phyllis, Holly, and Nicholas

AN IMPORTANT MESSAGE
FOR PARENTS

The contents of this book have been carefully chosen and arranged with a view toward helping parents evaluate those problems of infancy and childhood for which they might have to call their child's doctor. When used properly, this guide will assist in determining whether a child's condition or complaint is serious enough to require the doctor's immediate attention or advice.

The signs and symptoms of illnesses, injuries, and problems have been presented in their most usual and common course. When your child's condition differs from the description in this book, or appears to worsen despite a suggested treatment, or if you do not have a complete understanding of your child's problem, *always* call the doctor for additional discussion. It is better to make an "unnecessary" phone call than to risk having a serious illness go untreated. Whenever possible, discuss the contents of this book with your physician to be certain that its recommendations are similar to those which he or she would make to you.

PREFACE

Numerous child care guides are currently available which discuss illness, psychological problems, and well-baby care. In the past, only the most superficial attention has been given to one of the most important tools of communication used between parents and their physicians—the telephone. In fact, more than 20 percent of a practicing pediatrician's patient time may be spent dealing with problems over the telephone. Despite the essential nature of the telephone in communication between parents and their physicians, only recently have we examined the advantages, disadvantages, and ways of improving the quality of information which a patient receives over the telephone. Many parents consider the telephone a direct line which provides them with advice concerning their children, and it is not uncommon for many to respond to an acute illness by going directly from a hot forehead to the telephone.

During recent years, reliance on the telephone has increased because working mothers have less time to bring their children to the doctor, and borderline finances have forced many families to seek free telephone advice rather than pay for an office visit. In addition, as many families move from city to city, the pediatrician is often the person who provides advice to a new parent. My first book, *Telephone Medicine: A Practical Guide to Pediatric Telephone Advice* (St. Louis: C.V. Mosby Company, 1980), attempted to put in formal terms effective techniques for dealing with patients' concerns and medical problems over the telephone from the perspective of physicians and their assistants. It is unfortunate that most medical and nursing schools ignore telephone communications as a topic for teaching. Doctors and nurses are forced to learn how to deal with parents almost entirely on the job. This plight is not made easier when young parents, who are understandably inexperienced at asking questions to obtain the information that is important to them, give doctors or their assistants misleading or fuzzy clues as to what is happening with their children.

It is hoped that this book will provide much of the information usually supplied in standard child care manuals but with the orientation of helping parents to use the telephone properly when obtaining advice from their doctors concerning well-baby care and childhood illness.

This manual is not meant to be used in place of contacting a physician about medical matters. It is a guide containing useful information concerning the usual or common course of illnesses and symptoms.

Whenever your child's illness does not conform to this usual or common pattern or whenever you have an intuitive feeling that your child's problem is getting worse or is dangerous, always seek your doctor's advice for further instructions.

CONTENTS

Chapter I
BASIC PRINCIPLES OF USING THE TELEPHONE FOR CHILD CARE

Introduction
How to choose a doctor
Your doctor's receptionist
The doctor's office policy
Giving your complaint to the receptionist
The doctor's answering service
Talking with the doctor
How to make your doctor think you are
a terrific patient
Keeping notes
When to call the doctor
Getting medicines for your child
Leaving your child with babysitters
Your child's illness when you are away
from home
Emergency child care

1

USING THE TELEPHONE

COMMON COMPLAINTS

MINOR INFECTIONS

INFECTIOUS DISEASES

EMERGENCY PROBLEMS

NEW INFANT CARE

PEDIATRIC PROBLEMS

INTRODUCTION

Talking with your child's doctor, receptionist, office assistant, and answering service—when done properly—can save you time, money, and many unnecessary visits to the physician. For years these free telephone calls have been one of the best medical bargains in town. However, because of shyness, poor organization, and poor planning, many parents finish their telephone calls without receiving the information that is most important to them. More importantly, improper presentation of facts may mislead the doctor into giving them advice that is not accurate.

Understanding the workings of your doctor's office is essential to getting good medical care in general, but it is especially important for getting advice over the telephone. Treating non-emergencies as if they were urgent will eventually result in your doctor not believing you when a true crisis has arrived. Conversely, being too casual during an emergency situation may cause your child to suffer when he or she is not examined immediately.

HOW TO CHOOSE A DOCTOR

One of the most important decisions that you will ever have to make concerning your child's welfare will be choosing a doctor sympathetic to your problems and knowledgeable when offering medical advice. Availability for emergencies and acute problems should be a first priority when choosing a child's physician.

Information concerning doctors in your area can be obtained from neighborhood parents, and personnel from the local hospital. Although hospital personnel are often reluctant to recommend doctors by name, nursing staff and resident physicians may be willing to give the caller the names of one or two local physicians who respond to emergencies promptly and who have the reputation of being attentive to their patients' problems.

Physicians who have a pleasant personality, a large practice or a prestigious university appointment may not necessarily be the doctors who will provide you and your baby with availability, conscientiousness and knowledge when it is needed.

It is often helpful to contact the doctor's office to request that he meet with you for five or ten minutes to be sure that your personalities are compatible. A physician who is unwilling to comply with this reasonable request often will not be willing to see you during periods when you are under stress. If you believe that your attitudes concerning basic problems are not compatible, do not feel reluctant to interview other physi-

3

cians who will provide a pleasant relationship of many years' duration.

It is usually in your best interest to choose a physician who has a reputation for prescribing the fewest medicines possible and for suggesting diagnostic tests only when they are absolutely necessary. Many parents have the erroneous belief that they should take their child to the doctor so the doctor can give him something to relieve his symptoms or to treat his illness. It is unfortunate that many parents expect (and many doctors prescribe) antibiotics and other medicines for the most trivial illnesses. The complications from this overtreatment are often worse than the illness itself, which would have gotten better simply by waiting. The proper reason for bringing your child to the doctor for an examination is to make sure he will *not* be given medicines unless they are truly necessary for treating his specific illness.

Fever, colds, and simple coughs are not caused by a deficiency of antibiotics. When your physician cheerfully prescribes antibiotics for your child over the telephone (except in specific situations where he has an intimate knowledge of your child's condition), do not hesitate to ask him whether they are absolutely necessary. On the other hand, when your doctor spends additional time with you explaining why medicines are not necessary to treat a particular condition, do not pressure him to order medicines or tests simply because you feel anxious or nervous. It is not fair for your child to suffer the consequences of these unnecessary treatments because of someone else's poor judgment.

YOUR DOCTOR'S RECEPTIONIST

The person who answers the telephone in your child's doctor's office has an especially important role in helping both you and the physician. That individual is the person who screens telephone calls and determines whether they should be referred directly to the physician or charted to be answered at a later time. That person is usually also responsible for making appointments and helping the doctor arrange his time, and may influence your doctor's attitude toward your problem by the way that she presents it to him.

The receptionist has an especially difficult job because many parents feel nervous about calling their children's doctor. Their day is being disrupted, and they feel a tremendous sense of inconvenience and worry. They may therefore unknowingly release all of these frustrations when talking with the receptionist. She receives a constant barrage of "urgent" telephone calls and requests while receiving little praise for doing a good job.

4

If the receptionist sounds curt in her conversation with you, it may very well be the result of trying to do many jobs at the same time. She will usually be more responsive to those patients who talk in a friendly, pleasant manner and present her with accurate, concise information concerning their problems. This does not mean, however, that you should not be insistent when you believe that an emergency is not being given proper attention, but talking to the receptionist with an understanding of the difficulty of her job will provide you with many more favors over the long run than talking to her with disrespect.

THE DOCTOR'S OFFICE POLICY

At the time of your initial visit, many doctors' offices will provide patients with a printed sheet describing office policy. If this information is not provided, you will find it extremely helpful to request the following information and write it down for future reference:

1. Regular office hours:
   Weekdays:
   Weekends and holidays:
2. The best route to get to the office:
3. The usual fee schedule:
4. Office policy concerning insurance:
5. The usual intervals for routine physical examinations and immunizations:
6. What hospital emergency room does the physician prefer in the event that you have an emergency and what is its telephone number?
7. Does the doctor have a telephone calling hour? If not, during what hours would he prefer that you make your telephone calls?

USING THE TELEPHONE

COMMON COMPLAINTS

MINOR INFECTIONS

INFECTIOUS DISEASES

EMERGENCY PROBLEMS

NEW INFANT CARE

PEDIATRIC PROBLEMS

USING THE TELEPHONE

COMMON COMPLAINTS

MINOR INFECTIONS

INFECTIOUS DISEASES

EMERGENCY PROBLEMS

NEW INFANT CARE

PEDIATRIC PROBLEMS

GIVING YOUR COMPLAINT
TO THE RECEPTIONIST

Although most doctors develop the technique of returning a phone call to parents in a way that sounds as though it is the only call they have made that afternoon, many busy pediatricians return an average of four to six calls an hour, even during weekends. If these calls were all answered when they were phoned in, he would never have time to examine his patients or eat dinner. For that reason, many doctors instruct their receptionists and answering services to ask specific questions to sort out those patients who must be called back right away from those whose calls may wait until they can be returned as a group.

Once you are acquainted with your doctor's office procedures, don't waste time waiting for the doctor to call with information that can be given by office staff. Questions concerning billing, insurance, immunizations, frequency of checkups, etc., can almost always be answered by the office secretary. If you are reasonably certain that your child must be examined for his illness, tell the receptionist that you wish to make an appointment rather than asking her if you may speak with the doctor first. There is no reason to sit near the phone for a few hours only to be told something that you already know.

When you are talking to the doctor's secretary or answering service, do not give her a detailed story concerning the reason for the call. She does not need to know the history of your child's illness. Remember, her job is only to determine which calls should be put through to the doctor. It is therefore important to be certain that she understands whether your call is an emergency, whether it can be put off for a while, or whether it is related only to nonurgent information for which the doctor can call you back at his leisure.

Rule 1: Since some receptionists are not skilled at the job of screening questions, do not be timid when you talk with the receptionist. Tell her specifically how urgent or nonurgent your call is.

Examples of statements which accurately give information in brief terms to the receptionist are:
"This call is an emergency. My child has just hurt himself badly. Please get the doctor immediately."
"My child has a terrible earache. Please ask the doctor to call me as soon as possible."
"My child has a fever. I would like to talk to the doctor. When do you expect him to be making his calls next?"
"My child has a diaper rash. Please have the doctor call me when he has a chance."

Rule 2: In addition to telling the receptionist how urgent your message is, give her the following information *whether or not she asks for it*:

    (a) The name and age of your child

    (b) A one- or two-sentence description of his illness (Johnny has a cold/fever/rash/chicken pox).

    (c) The telephone number where you can be reached and how long you will be there ("I will be at 555-1000 until three, then I will be at 555-2000").

Rule 3: If you do not receive a call from your doctor within a reasonable period of time, *call his office back*. He may truly have been unable to call you because he was not immediately available or because he was out on an emergency. But in a busy office a message may occasionally be misplaced, your phone number may have been taken incorrectly, or the urgency of the message may have not been noted appropriately. Calling back may save you undue anxiety and prevent misunderstandings.

THE DOCTOR'S ANSWERING SERVICE

Most acute-care physicians have a telephone answering service to take messages when they are not in the office. The majority of these operators are friendly and efficient in taking information, but remember that most have no formal training in medical matters. Do not ask the answering service operator for medical advice concerning illnesses or other problems but reserve these questions specifically for your physician or his office staff.

As with your physician's secretary or receptionist, answering service operators have to sort calls concerning their degree of urgency, and it is the operator's responsibility to determine whether or not a physician must be contacted on an urgent basis.

In addition to telling the operator where he will be during a given period of time, your doctor will usually tell the operator when he next expects to be calling in to pick up routine telephone messages. It can be extremely helpful to you if you ask when she expects the doctor to call in, since this will give you some idea of whether it is necessary to disturb him earlier. If your physician has just contacted his service at 1:00 P.M. and is expected to call in at 3:30 P.M., your 1:15 P.M. call may not be able to

7

USING THE TELEPHONE

COMMON COMPLAINTS

MINOR INFECTIONS

INFECTIOUS DISEASES

EMERGENCY PROBLEMS

NEW INFANT CARE

PEDIATRIC PROBLEMS

wait that long. On the other hand, if you are calling at 3:15 P.M., there is no reason to disturb him sooner.

Because answering service operators do not uniformly use good judgment, leave nothing to their imagination concerning the urgency of your call. If you believe that it is a true emergency, say so. If you believe that the call is not urgent, tell her specifically that the doctor should call you when he calls in next.

TALKING WITH THE DOCTOR

When you call your child's doctor, you want to be certain that when you hang up the telephone you have the information that you really wanted and that you understand what the doctor told you. This sounds so obvious as not to deserve mention, but it is surprising how many parents have such difficulty in organizing their thoughts that the doctor honestly cannot tell the real reason for the call. Many of the usual problems in communication can be avoided by following these basic principles.

Rule 1. Introduce yourself properly.

"This is Mrs. Preston. I am calling about my daughter, Susie, who is three years old."

Age information may not be necessary for a doctor who has examined your child regularly, but there is no reason to take the chance that she may be confused with a sibling or with a child who has a similar name.

Rule 2. Tell the doctor the *real* reason for the telephone call.

"Susie only has a cold but I need to know if my mother, who will be visiting, can catch it."

"The baby seems to have a cold, but my neighbor's baby has pneumonia. Should I be concerned?"

"Margaret has another cold but doesn't look terribly sick. This is her third cold in four weeks. Should I be concerned about the frequent illnesses?"

When you don't tell the doctor the actual reason that you are calling, you may not find out the information that you really want to know, or else the doctor may be curt because your question sounds so trivial. In the first two cases, if you called the doctor after hours to ask if the cold is contagious or to tell him that the baby has a runny nose but doesn't look sick, it would be easy to misinterpret these calls as being trivial or a nuisance. However, if you follow the rule of telling the doctor specifically why you are concerned, that after-hours call will make more

8

sense. In the third example, if you do not let the doctor know that you are troubled by the frequency of the colds rather than by this particular cold, you will probably be given a lecture on using a decongestant rather than a discussion about recurrent illnesses.

Rule 3. *Give the most important information first.*

The section of this book which deals with symptoms tells you what the doctor needs to know about your child's complaint or illness. But tell the doctor the most important information first, beginning with what is happening now rather than what happened two weeks ago. When you tell the doctor that "My child has had a painful earache for one hour and has just begun having fever" you have given the most important information first. Without further discussion, the doctor may tell you that it is necessary to have your youngster examined or he may tell you what to do to relieve symptoms. It is not necessary to explain that Johnny has had a cold for one week, had a fever three days ago which went away, had exposure to cousins who have strep throat, and that he hasn't looked right all winter. The most important information is that he has an earache and fever *now*. The other information may also be important to your doctor, but it is not the primary concern.

Rule 4. *Be brief.*

Your time is valuable. So is the doctor's. Don't waste either with unnecessary conversation.

Rule 5. *Understand what was said.*

If your doctor gives you information that is difficult to understand, say "I'm sorry but I don't understand what you just told me." Many parents try to bluff their way through these common situations either because they feel embarrassed or because they feel that their doctor is in a hurry. Where your child's health is concerned, these reasons are absolutely ridiculous. More often than not, the fault is not yours and most doctors do not mind making a second explanation using different words. Moreover, it is most likely that if the information is important, you will have to call the doctor back anyway.

COMMON COMPLAINTS

MINOR INFECTIONS

INFECTIOUS DISEASES

EMERGENCY PROBLEMS

NEW INFANT CARE

PEDIATRIC PROBLEMS

9

USING THE
TELEPHONE

COMMON
COMPLAINTS

MINOR
INFECTIONS

INFECTIOUS
DISEASES

EMERGENCY
PROBLEMS

NEW INFANT
CARE

PEDIATRIC
PROBLEMS

HOW TO MAKE YOUR DOCTOR THINK YOU ARE A TERRIFIC PATIENT

1. Call your doctor during regular hours.

Most children's doctors have a calling hour or times during the day that are preferred for making non-emergency calls. If you are not certain when these times are, ask your doctor's secretary. It is simply not fair to bother your doctor with an after-hours telephone call to obtain information when no emergency exists. Doctors will sometimes joke among themselves that when patients say "I am using Dr. Smith," they mean it quite literally.

Those doctors who are friendly and take a strong personal interest in their patients run the risk of being called for minor complaints after hours because parents think that he or she would want to know about their child's minor injury or illness. Physicians often become formal with parents who think of them as a twenty-four-hour service which may be called at any time. Regardless of their personalities, however, all doctors would prefer to be called about routine matters during office hours.

2. Acknowledge an inconvenience.

Doctors are regular people with families. They try to eat uninterrupted meals and like to get to bed at a reasonable hour. If it is necessary to call your physician after regular hours, you can make him much more receptive to your call. Simply acknowledge the fact that you are interrupting his privacy, by saying "Sorry to call you so late, but . . ." or "I'm sorry that I couldn't have called earlier, but . . ." These remarks let the doctor know that you regard him as a person rather than as a machine.

It is not difficult to understand why he would feel disgruntled by an 11:00 P.M. caller who presents information as though it were the middle of the afternoon. "Hi, Dr. Smith. My two-year-old Johnny just woke up with a cough. What medicine do you think I should give him?" At the extreme, doctors with office phones in their homes frequently gripe about patients who call at 2:00 A.M. and upon hearing the doctor's voice say "Oh, Dr. Smith, are you in the office now?"

Your apology represents good manners but, more importantly, it decreases the chance that your doctor may respond gruffly simply because of the timing of your call.

10

3. Avoid ambiguity.

When a physician receives an emergency page while he is in his car, at a movie, or at dinner, and finds that the emergency was really a routine telephone call, it is often difficult for him to be polite to the caller. If you tell his answering service operator that "the baby is having trouble breathing" when he has a stuffy nose, or that your child "has bloody diarrhea" when you notice a single strand of bloody mucus, the disruption of your doctor's activities is obviously not justified. If you cannot avoid presenting your child's symptoms in a way that makes a non-emergency sound like an emergency, simply tell the answering service operator or receptionist that the call is not urgent.

4. Don't panic for non-emergencies.

Most physicians understand that some parents are more disturbed than other parents by their child's illnesses. These parents may truly run the risk that when their child develops a problem requiring immediate attention, they may not receive it after three previous calls for non-emergency emergencies.

If you know that it is difficult for you to tell when something is an emergency, tell the doctor exactly that and allow him to make the determination for you. "I'm sorry to bother you, Doctor, but I honestly was frightened by Johnny's fever. Should I worry about it and if not, when should I be concerned?"

In summary, the best way to get an understanding response from your doctor is to treat him with the same courtesy used toward any other person. When problems are non-emergencies, try to contact him or her during regular hours. If you reach a secretary or answering service, tell them specifically that the call is not an emergency. Emergency calls, on the other hand, should be treated as if they require immediate attention. Don't be embarrassed about asking for it.

KEEPING NOTES

Many parents find it reassuring to contact their physician each time the child has a cold, even though they expect to be given exactly the same information that they were given two or three weeks before. "Checking in" with your doctor each time your child becomes ill is usually not necessary unless there is some element to the illness which was not previously present.

Keeping a small notebook in which to record your doctor's preferred

COMMON COMPLAINTS

MINOR INFECTIONS

INFECTIOUS DISEASES

EMERGENCY PROBLEMS

NEW INFANT CARE

PEDIATRIC PROBLEMS

11

USING THE TELEPHONE

COMMON COMPLAINTS

MINOR INFECTIONS

INFECTIOUS DISEASES

EMERGENCY PROBLEMS

NEW INFANT CARE

PEDIATRIC PROBLEMS

medicines for routine illness and the dosage which he has recommended will save both you and your doctor wasted time. It will also gradually help you to feel more secure in dealing with your child's illness.

During actual conversations with your doctor, have a pencil and paper next to the telephone to record information as he gives it to you. There is no more frustrating experience for either a doctor or a parent than to have a telephone conversation which discusses medicines, dosage, and advice at length, only to realize that little of it was remembered because of nervousness, distraction, or difficulty with language.

WHEN TO CALL THE DOCTOR

Because taking care of children is such an important responsibility, many parents are so afraid of making a mistake that they rely almost totally on the advice of others before making a decision. It is not unusual for pediatricians to deal with parents who ask them questions concerning even minor aspects of their children's lives, including schooling, socializing with friends, proper clothing for winter and summer wear, length of time their children can remain in the tub, etc.

Much of this insecurity is caused by articles in the media stressing the hidden dangers of "improper" child rearing, food additives, environmental pollutants, and education. At the same time, stories are presented and experts are interviewed who always advise parents of the "best" way to raise or care for their children. It is not surprising that many parents will therefore be anxious about matters that concern their child's health.

The most important tool parents have that will allow them to care for their children so as to make few major mistakes is their *intuitive feeling* as to whether what they are doing is "correct." Educating oneself about medical and psychological matters is important, but not at the expense of intuition and common sense.

When your child has a high fever but does not look particularly ill, the likelihood of a serious illness is slight. When your child has no fever or specific complaints, but looks "toxic," is difficult to arouse, and generally looks as though he is very sick, he probably is. When your child is a "terrible eater" but looks well nourished, his nutrition cannot be terribly bad. If you worry about the friends that your child is making, that he is not doing his best in school, and that your relationship with him is not going as well as you would like, but he generally seems happy and his teacher says that his work is satisfactory, it is not likely that he has any major problems. However, if you cannot find any one specific difficulty he is having but he seems depressed most of the time, you will probably be right in assuming that there really is something bothering him.

Using "experts" such as your physician to answer questions about health, illness, and behavior can be very helpful and should be carefully considered when raising your children, but *never* stop using your own intuitive feelings or common sense. When someone tells you that something is right or wrong, it generally is true in most cases, but may not be the best advice in this particular instance or for your family situation.

Call your doctor if you have been managing a problem which is not improving, or if you do not have adequate information to make an important decision. When you believe that something is an emergency, it *is* an emergency to you. If you feel reassured after talking to the doctor, follow his advice accurately. If your intuition tells you that the problem has not been solved, or if you believe that an emergency still exists, call the doctor back to be certain that there were no misunderstandings.

If an error is to be made, always make it in the direction of being overcautious. While we have tried to make the advice in this manual as accurate as possible, you are the only one who is actually looking at your child when a problem arises. When you believe that your child's appearance is especially poor; if his general level of activity makes him appear "lifeless" or lethargic; if he looks apprehensive or very pale; if he looks much sicker than he usually does when he becomes ill, he should be considered *toxic*. This single consideration should outweigh all others when prompting you to call your doctor on an emergency basis.

GETTING MEDICINES
FOR YOUR CHILD

Since medicines have become so expensive in recent years, comparison shopping for prices has become a routine procedure for many parents. Discount pharmacies may dispense prescriptions at relatively low prices. A small neighborhood pharmacy, on the other hand, usually provides more personalized attention, allows you to charge merchandise, and many will deliver medicines to your home. The cost of buying medicines at local pharmacies is higher because these additional services will substantially increase your pharmacist's overhead and he, of course, will pass it on to you.

Many parents will shop in both places but it is a major convenience to maintain an active charge account at a pharmacy that will keep accessible records concerning past prescriptions, record allergies that your

13

COMMON COMPLAINTS

MINOR INFECTIONS

INFECTIOUS DISEASES

EMERGENCY PROBLEMS

NEW INFANT CARE

PEDIATRIC PROBLEMS

child may have developed, and after receiving a phone call from your physician, will deliver medicine directly to your home when you cannot make the trip yourself. Introduce yourself to your pharmacist, try to develop a personal relationship with him, and give him the respect he deserves for being an important asset to the community.

LEAVING YOUR CHILD
WITH BABYSITTERS

Much of the information described in this chapter—information concerning your doctor's telephone number, the best time to call, common medicines with their dosages, and the place to take your child in case of an emergency—should be left within easy access of a babysitter whether she is a teenager, a professional, or a relative. Most medical decisions are best made by your doctor rather than by a babysitter. Leaving his or her telephone number is usually adequate, but the other information may prove extremely useful. When you are leaving your child in the care of another person for a prolonged period of time as you might when going on a vacation, it is wise to leave the babysitter with a note stating:

"In the event of a medical emergency which involves my children named———, I hereby delegate———to take legal responsibility for decisions concerning their medical well-being should I not be available to give my consent." Signed———Date———

In most instances, your child's doctor will assume responsibility for medical care if you have been his regular patient. Although surgical problems and medical emergencies do not commonly occur during periods when you cannot be reached, planning for this possibility increases the probability that your child will get proper medical care without undue delay.

YOUR CHILD'S ILLNESS
WHEN YOU ARE AWAY FROM HOME

If your child becomes ill while you are on vacation or visiting with friends or relatives, you may save yourself much anxiety and time by telephoning your regular child's doctor from out of town instead of trying to seek local medical help. Although calling a New York doctor from Chicago might not first come to mind when your child is sick, there will

COMMON COMPLAINTS

MINOR INFECTIONS

INFECTIOUS DISEASES

EMERGENCY PROBLEMS

NEW INFANT CARE

PEDIATRIC PROBLEMS

be many times when your own doctor may be able to advise you of proper medical care over the telephone.

Many out-of-town pharmacists will accept prescriptions from out-of-state physicians for medicines which do not contain narcotics or tranquilizers. In addition, your own doctor may also be able to advise you of those illnesses for which an immediate examination of your child by a local physician is absolutely necessary.

If the problem cannot be solved over the telephone, a physician referral may be obtained from your friends or relatives, or from the hotel at which you are staying. Many hotel managers keep lists of recommended physicians and specialists for this purpose. When rapid attention is necessary, however, bring your child directly to the nearest hospital emergency room even though you might not use an emergency room for a similar illness if you were at home. Parents who frequently travel with their children have told us that they have developed the practice of asking for travel instructions to the nearest hospital as part of their travel plans whenever they are staying in a new location for any prolonged period of time.

EMERGENCY
CHILD CARE

When an emergency occurs during your doctor's regular office hours, always telephone that number first to ask for advice. During non-office hours, if you believe the situation to be life-threatening or requiring immediate medical attention, bring your child directly to the emergency facility your doctor has recommended and leave a message with his answering service that you are en route to the hospital. If you are feeling too nervous to drive safely, call a neighbor or the police department rather than an ambulance for more rapid transportation. Because most children can be transported easily in one's arms, a police car with a rapid response time may be more beneficial than an ambulance that contains more emergency equipment, but often has a longer response time. Consult your doctor for advice since conditions vary in different locations.

15

USING THE TELEPHONE

COMMON COMPLAINTS

MINOR INFECTIONS

INFECTIOUS DISEASES

EMERGENCY PROBLEMS

NEW INFANT CARE

PEDIATRIC PROBLEMS

Chapter II
COMMON SYMPTOMATIC COMPLAINTS

Fever
Colds (upper respiratory infections)
Sore throat (pharyngitis)
Earache (otitis)
Cough
Wheezing (asthma, asthmatic bronchitis)
Croup (barking cough)
Nosebleed (epistaxis)
Headache
Stomach pain in older children
Stomach pain (including colic) in infants
Vomiting (emesis)
Diarrhea
Constipation
Pain on urination (dysuria)
Rashes (not including diaper rash)
Diaper rash

USING THE TELEPHONE

COMMON COMPLAINTS

MINOR INFECTIONS

INFECTIOUS DISEASES

EMERGENCY PROBLEMS

NEW INFANT CARE

PEDIATRIC PROBLEMS

USING THE TELEPHONE

COMMON COMPLAINTS

MINOR INFECTIONS

INFECTIOUS DISEASES

EMERGENCY PROBLEMS

NEW INFANT CARE

PEDIATRIC PROBLEMS

FEVER

What the doctor needs to know:

1. *Age:* How old is your child?
2. *Fever:* How high is the fever and how long has it been present?
3. *Other Symptoms:* Have you noticed other symptoms such as running nose, pulling at ears, cough, vomiting, diarrhea, or rash? (See each symptom section.)
4. *Pain:* Has your child complained of pain in his throat, ears, stomach, or head?
5. *General Condition:* How does your child look when you compare this illness with others she's had?

Call the doctor immediately if:

1. The fever is greater than 105°F (40.6°C) after fever-lowering medication has been given.
2. Your youngster looks and acts extremely sick, i.e., she is difficult to arouse, speaks without making sense or generally appears toxic after fever-lowering medication has been given. (See pages 12–13, "When To Call the Doctor.")
3. Your intuitive feeling tells you that your child is very sick.

Call the doctor in the near future if:

1. Your child's fever is greater than 101°F (38.4°C) for more than 24 hours.
2. Her fever comes and goes but other symptoms are present for more than three days.

Treatment of fever

1. If your child has fever and appears ill, give aspirin (one baby aspirin for each fifteen pounds of body weight) or an aspirin substitute (follow directions on the label) every 3 to 4 hours. Feel your youngster fifteen minutes later. If she is still hot, take her temperature. If it is more than 104°F (40°C) and she feels

USING THE TELEPHONE

COMMON COMPLAINTS

MINOR INFECTIONS

INFECTIOUS DISEASES

EMERGENCY PROBLEMS

NEW INFANT CARE

PEDIATRIC PROBLEMS

19

USING THE
TELEPHONE

COMMON
COMPLAINTS

MINOR
INFECTIONS

INFECTIOUS
DISEASES

EMERGENCY
PROBLEMS

NEW INFANT
CARE

PEDIATRIC
PROBLEMS

uncomfortable, place her in a bath filled with lukewarm water for fifteen minutes.

2. Dress your child in loose-fitting, lightweight cotton clothing to absorb perspiration, and cover her lightly. If she has chills or complains of being cold, cover her with a blanket only during that short period of time. The room temperature is best kept toward the cool side. In the summer, an air conditioner is helpful.

3. Feed your child soft bland foods. If she refuses these, offer clear liquids. Water alone should be avoided since it contains no calories.

4. Arrange to have your youngster examined if her illness continues or gets worse.

Discussion:

Although fever is a frequent sign of illness and may often be found in children who do not appear very ill, many parents become frightened just because it is present. Most pediatricians now agree that unless the fever is greater than 107°F it is unlikely to be associated with any long-term damage to your child. In general, the height of the fever is a very poor guide to the degree of illness in youngsters. We are much more concerned about a child with a temperature of 101°F (38.4°C) who is difficult to arouse and appears very lethargic than about one who has a temperature of 105°F (40.6°C) and is leaping around in her crib. The presence or absence of fever may be useful in determining whether a well-appearing child may be sick or for following the course of an illness but has little other value.

There is a growing trend among pediatricians not to treat an elevated temperature unless the patient is uncomfortable. Their feeling is that the body produces fever (by causing chills or increased muscle tension resulting in muscle aches) as a helpful mechanism to aid the body in fighting off germs. According to this theory, when you give aspirin to lower the temperature, it may be the equivalent of giving a patient a drug to lower his white blood cell count when it is found to be elevated. This would make the laboratory test appear normal, but would certainly not be in the patient's best interest. This nontreatment practice is often followed in the hospital by most physicians where aspirin and sponge bathing are only given for very high temperature and for relief of discomfort.

When the illness is not severe, it is wise to allow your child to have a fever (temperature less than 101°F (38.4°C) has no significance) for twenty-four hours or more before requesting that the doctor examine her. This will screen out those illnesses which are caused by short "twenty-four-hour viruses." After this period, an infected ear or throat may have developed and will be observed by your physician upon examination. At an earlier time these findings may not have been present.

Do not be afraid to bring your child to the doctor's office when she has a fever. It is reasonable to assume that if undressing your child, bathing her in lukewarm water, and keeping her in a cool room are useful methods of lowering her temperature, taking her outside will not be harmful. It is also for these reasons that giving your child a bath or washing her hair when she is sick will not make the illness worse and may improve her disposition. Going to the doctor's office also has the advantage of allowing an examination with optimal conditions.

Alcohol rubs have little advantage over tepid bathing and should especially be avoided in an unventilated room. Prolonged exposure to the alcohol vapors may cause alcohol intoxication in small children and may cause the blood sugar to drop to dangerously low levels.

Fever convulsions are mentioned only to explain that they are uncommon when compared with the total number of high fevers that children have and are rarely seen below the age of one year or over the age of five years. They are more common when there has been a family history of fever convulsions and are usually seen when the fever has its initial rise. Most importantly, simple fever convulsions rarely, if ever, cause brain damage unless they are associated with a central nervous system infection like meningitis. Convulsions commonly give the parents of the child a terrible scare, but the children do very well (usually without any treatment). Management of these fever convulsions is discussed in Chapter VI, "Emergency Problems."

In summary, fever is a body response to infection that is probably more useful than it is harmful. It should be treated with aspirin or similar anti-fever medicines, tepid sponging, and cool environment when your child feels uncomfortable. The source of the infection should be searched for by your doctor if your child looks very sick or if the fever has been greater than 101°F (38.4°C) for more than one day. Bringing your youngster to the doctor's office may not always be convenient, but it is not harmful to him. It also assures your child of an examination with proper lighting, diagnostic tools, and available medication.

21

USING THE
TELEPHONE

COMMON
COMPLAINTS

MINOR
INFECTIONS

INFECTIOUS
DISEASES

EMERGENCY
PROBLEMS

NEW INFANT
CARE

PEDIATRIC
PROBLEMS

COLDS
(UPPER RESPIRATORY INFECTIONS)

What the doctor needs to know:

1. *Age:* How old is your child?
2. *Duration:* How long has he had the cold?
3. *Fever:* If there is fever, how high is it? How long has it been present? Is it constant or does it come and go?
4. *Nasal discharge:* Does the discharge from your child's nose have a greenish-yellow color that looks like pus?
5. *Cough:* If your child has a cough, does it occur only at night and in the early morning, or does it continue all through the day?
6. *Pain:* Does your child complain of severe throat or ear pain?
7. *General appearance:* Does your child appear reasonably well, or does he look sicker than he usually looks when he has a cold?

Call the doctor immediately if:

Your child appears very ill and you are concerned about his general appearance. (See pages 12–13, "When to call the Doctor.")

Call the doctor in the near future if:

1. Your child's cold has lasted longer than ten days.
2. He has had a continuous temperature of more than 101˚F (38.4˚C) for more than twenty-four hours.
3. The youngster has had a discharge from his nose that looks like pus or has had a sore throat for more than two days.
4. Your child has a cough that persists all day for more than twenty-four hours, especially if it has a short, dry, repeating quality or is associated with wheezing.

Treatment for infants less than six months old:

1. Place two or three drops of normal saline (salt water) solution in your baby's nose before feedings and at bedtime. These drops may be purchased at the pharmacy without a prescription.
2. If the baby's nose is actively running, the mucus may be removed with a nasal suction bulb syringe.
3. A vaporizer may be placed next to your baby's bedside if he is breathing through his mouth. Do not place medication in the vaporizer.
4. The head-end of your baby's crib should be propped up by placing books under the legs of the crib.

Treatment for children more than six months old:

1. Decongestants may be given in the dosage suggested on the bottle or by your physician.
2. A vaporizer may be placed next to your child's bedside, especially if he is breathing through his mouth. No medication should be added to the vaporizer.
3. Your child may be given a cough suppressant at night if the cough is preventing sleep.

Discussion

When pediatricians ask themselves why parents call them so frequently about simple colds, they have often forgotten how pathetic a small baby looks when he is trying to breathe through a stuffed nose and is having trouble sleeping and eating. They may also forget that when parents are not certain whether older children can go to school, babysitters must be arranged for, numerous plans have to be changed, and some parents may have to remain home from their jobs.

There is often additional frustration because many children seem to get colds so frequently that they almost always appear sick. This is especially true since children who are nursery school and kindergarten age may average eight to ten colds per year. When each cold lasts one or one and a half weeks and there is a three-day interval between colds, two colds in sequence can cause three weeks of illness. This is a very long time to watch your child's nose running and to listen to him cough at

23

USING THE
TELEPHONE

COMMON
COMPLAINTS

MINOR
INFECTIONS

INFECTIOUS
DISEASES

EMERGENCY
PROBLEMS

NEW INFANT
CARE

PEDIATRIC
PROBLEMS

night without becoming concerned over a possibly more serious underlying illness.

If your child has had a fever of more than 101°F for longer than one day, he should be evaluated by his doctor to be certain that he does not have a secondary bacterial infection such as bronchitis or a streptococcal throat infection. Similarly, persistence of green or yellow discharge from the nose may indicate an infection in your youngster's ears or sinuses. Also, a cough that is present throughout the day may be caused by bronchitis or pneumonia.

If your child's temperature or pussy nasal discharge comes and goes, it has no real significance and may be present throughout the seven to ten days of the cold. When the cough occurs only at night and in the early morning, it is also of little importance since it usually reflects a discharge of mucus going down the back of his throat when he lies flat.

When your child is small, the safest medicine to use is normal saline (salt water) nose drops. Place these drops in the baby's nose before feedings to make it easier for him to suck and breathe at the same time. Because of breathing through the mouth and increased swallowing of air, many babies will spit more or become more gassy when they have a cold.

Older children with cold symptoms may have some relief when they take decongestants. Over-the-counter preparations and prescription drugs contain similar medicines and there is little advantage to having five varieties in the house at the same time. Watch your children for signs of irritability or sleepiness while they are taking these medicines. These symptoms are often thought to be the result of the cold when they are actually being caused by the medicine. Decongestant nose drops are occasionally of value, but most children do not like to have them inserted. Also, if the drops are used over a long period of time, they may cause *increased* nasal stuffiness because of "rebound" irritation to the lining of the nose.

Vaporizers have been very popular through the years but they never have been proven to be very effective. They are useful for relief of a dry throat if your child is breathing with his mouth open because of a stuffed nose, but having the paint or wallpaper peeling from your child's bedroom walls may be more of a nuisance than it is worth. Adding medication to the vaporizer water should be avoided since it may act as an irritant to your child's air passages, especially if he is an infant. A white coating to the tongue may also be noted because of mouth breathing which allows the cells which cover the tongue to accumulate.

Most important to managing your child's cold is awareness of his general condition as an overall guide to whether his illness is getting better or worse. Because none of the medications will shorten the course

24

of his illness but merely provide some relief of symptoms, give your child medication only when he is disturbed by his symptoms—not when you don't like the way he sounds. Many undesirable side effects can be avoided this way, and it is much easier to keep the illness in its proper perspective.

In summary, most colds have an uncomplicated course of seven to ten days but may appear to last longer when they occur in sequence. Any symptom that is persistent and appears to be worsening should be evaluated by the doctor. Medication should be given to the child only when he has symptoms disturbing to him, but remember that the medications may have side effects that may make your youngster appear to be getting worse.

Additional information may be found in the sections on Fever (p. 19), Cough (p. 32), Earache (p. 29), and Sore Throat (p. 26).

USING THE TELEPHONE

COMMON COMPLAINTS

MINOR INFECTIONS

INFECTIOUS DISEASES

EMERGENCY PROBLEMS

NEW INFANT CARE

PEDIATRIC PROBLEMS

USING THE
TELEPHONE

COMMON
COMPLAINTS

MINOR
INFECTIONS

INFECTIOUS
DISEASES

EMERGENCY
PROBLEMS

NEW INFANT
CARE

PEDIATRIC
PROBLEMS

SORE THROAT
(PHARYNGITIS)

What the doctor needs to know:

1. *Age:* How old is your child?
2. *Pain:* Is the throat very painful or is it a minor complaint?
3. *Fever:* If your child has fever, how high is it and how long has it been present?
4. *Cold:* Does your child also have a cold or hoarseness?
5. *Swollen glands:* Is there a tender swelling in the neck?
6. *Exposure:* Has your child recently been exposed to other youngsters with streptococcal infections?
7. *Rash:* Does your child have a sandpapery rash over his body which is more severe in the groin and under the arms?
8. *Breathing difficulty:* Does your child have difficulty with his breathing, or drooling from the mouth?
9. *General condition:* Does your child appear well or does he look especially ill?

Call the doctor immediately if:

1. The child appears especially sick. (See pages 12–13, "When to Call the Doctor.")
2. Your child has a rash.
3. Your child has severe difficulty with breathing or drooling from the mouth.

Call the doctor in the near future if:

1. Your youngster has a temperature of more than 101˚F (38.4˚C) for more than 24 hours, especially if the fever is not lowered by aspirin.
2. There is tender swelling in the neck.
3. There has been recent exposure to streptococcal infection.
4. You have been advised that there is a high incidence of streptococcal infection in your child's school or neighborhood.
5. Throat pain has been present for more than three days.

Treatment:

1. Give aspirin or acetaminophen if your child has fever or severe discomfort.
2. Throat lozenges, sucking candy, or honey are useful to relieve throat pain.

Discussion:

Sore throat or pharyngitis, a complaint common to many colds, often can be relieved by coating the back of the throat with a layer of sugar found in honey, throat lozenges, or sucking candy. Throat pain usually causes only minor discomfort and does not have a major significance. However, streptococcal infections of the throat (strep throat) have been associated with rheumatic fever, which can cause heart disease and kidney disease (glomerulonephritis). Therefore, diagnosing these youngsters and treating them with antibiotics, such as penicillin, is of major importance. Parents should know, however, that the likelihood of complications developing from streptococcal sore throat is really very small. One of the major advantages of early treatment of strep throat is the prevention of the spread of illness to friends and brothers and sisters of these children.

Although some signs of infection make the diagnosis of strep throat more likely (hemorrhages in the back of the throat, tender swelling in the neck, and fever not relieved by aspirin), these physical findings are often not reliable in making a diagnosis. The only way your doctor can make an accurate diagnosis of strep throat is by taking a throat culture. Knowing whether there is a high incidence of streptococcal infection in your community or in your child's school is especially important because when the incidence is high, your child should have a throat culture taken early in the course of the disease. When the incidence is low, it's reasonable to wait through two or three days of illness before visiting the doctor, unless your child looks especially sick.

If your child has a cold or hoarseness (laryngitis), these symptoms usually indicate a viral infection which will not normally respond to antibiotics. However, when the symptoms continue for more than a few days, you should ask your doctor's advice. If your youngster has a sore throat and develops a sandpapery rash that is present over most of his body but is especially noticeable in the creases under the arms or in the groin, scarlet fever should be suspected. In the case of an older child who has difficulty with breathing or is drooling, the possibility that he may be developing an abscess or a boil in the back of his throat should prompt

USING THE TELEPHONE

COMMON COMPLAINTS

MINOR INFECTIONS

INFECTIOUS DISEASES

EMERGENCY PROBLEMS

NEW INFANT CARE

PEDIATRIC PROBLEMS

27

you to contact your physician immediately. Drooling has little significance in small children, however.

In summary, most sore throats are minor and are the result of colds or upper respiratory tract infections. It is necessary to contact your physician on an emergency basis only if you have an older child who has a rash suggestive of scarlet fever, who appears toxic or especially sick, or who is having true difficulty with his breathing. Because of the possibility that the symptoms may be caused by streptococcal infection, your physician should be contacted on a non-urgent basis to determine whether he believes that a throat culture is necessary for diagnosis. Medications that do not require a prescription are usually successful for relieving symptoms, and a vaporizer may be useful on occasion when your child is breathing through his mouth.

Additional information may be found in the sections on Fever (p. 19) and Colds (p. 22).

28

EARACHE
(OTITIS)

What the doctor needs to know:

1. *Age:* How old is your child?
2. *Duration:* How long has she complained of an earache?
3. *Fever:* If your child has fever, how long has it been present and how high is it?
4. *Pain:* Does your child have minor pain or is it especially severe?
5. *Cold:* Does your child also have sore throat or cold?
6. *Discharge:* Is there a discharge from the ear?
7. *External pain:* Does it hurt when you press on the button-like structure in front of the ear?
8. *General condition:* Does your child look toxic or especially sick at this time?

Call the doctor immediately if:

1. The child appears toxic or especially ill. (See pages 12–13, "When to Call the Doctor.")
2. Your child has severe pain lasting longer than one hour not relieved with the suggested remedies.

Call the doctor in the near future if:

1. Your youngster has ear pain lasting longer than one hour even if the symptoms disappear without treatment.
2. There is a temperature higher than 101°F. (38.4°C).
3. Ear discharge is present.

Treatment:

1. Aspirin, acetaminophen, or other pain relievers should be given by mouth and anesthetic eardrops may be used if they are available.
2. Cold medicines containing decongestants may be useful.
3. Heat may be applied to the ear using a heating pad or warm washcloth.

USING THE TELEPHONE

COMMON COMPLAINTS

MINOR INFECTIONS

INFECTIOUS DISEASES

EMERGENCY PROBLEMS

NEW INFANT CARE

PEDIATRIC PROBLEMS

USING THE
TELEPHONE

COMMON
COMPLAINTS

MINOR
INFECTIONS

INFECTIOUS
DISEASES

EMERGENCY
PROBLEMS

NEW INFANT
CARE

PEDIATRIC
PROBLEMS

4. Most children will be more comfortable when placed in a sitting rather than lying-down position.
5. Be very reassuring when talking with your youngster since many children are frightened when they have pain.

Discussion:

Ear infections are generally of two types. The one that is referred to as swimmer's ear (external otitis) is actually a skin infection of the ear canal. This occurs more commonly during the summer months and can often be diagnosed at home if pain is present when finger pressure is applied to the small button (the tragus) in front of the ear. Sometimes pain can also be elicited by pulling with gentle pressure on the outer portion of the ear. When there is a strong suspicion that swimmer's ear is present, your physician may prescribe eardrops that contain either a vinegar-like solution or antibiotics and that may be applied a few times a day. Heat and aspirin are also useful in relieving the symptoms. To prevent further irritation, children should avoid getting water in their ear canals for at least a one-week period. If swimming or bathing cannot be avoided, ear plugs may be made using pieces of cotton covered with a petroleum jelly, such as Vaseline.

The more common type of ear infection is one which affects the middle ear (otitis media). The usual story we hear from parents whose children have this type of infection is that the child has had a cold for two or three days, lies down for a nap or in preparation for sleep, and is awakened two to three hours later with severe ear pain that lasts four to eight hours. Often the child will fall asleep again and awaken in the morning with only mild symptoms or none at all. Because this middle-ear infection is present *behind* the eardrum, eardrops are of no value for treatment. Once he is certain of the diagnosis, your physician will usually prescribe antibiotics to be given either by mouth or by injection. Ear pain will often be relieved by using analgesics such as aspirin or acetaminophen. Medicines containing codeine are often especially helpful and the application of heat may provide some temporary relief. While the symptoms of earache will usually disappear within a few hours without the help of medications, your physician should be contacted even though your child may have improved remarkably without any treatment. Since the infection rests behind the eardrum rather than in front of it, avoidance of bathing or swimming is not usually necessary although deep-water diving may cause discomfort because of the change in pressure. Similarly, flying in an airplane may cause pain or rupture of the eardrum.

If your child has an ear discharge with only minor pain, your physician should still be contacted on a nonurgent basis because the discharge may represent pus that is leaking through the eardrum, or it may be the result of wax that has melted because of the heat generated by the infected eardrum. In either case, when ear discharge has been noted, medicine should not be placed in the ear without the approval of your physician, because if the eardrum has been punctured these drops may find their way into the middle ear causing damage.

In summary, swimmer's ear (external otitis) is a skin infection of the ear canal that is more common in the summer months and that is suggested by pain caused when pressure is put on the outer part of the ear. Earaches caused by an infection of the middle ear (otitis media) are of special importance because they can be adequately treated only by using prescription antibiotics that are taken internally. Your physician should be contacted for advice on a nonurgent basis, even if the earache disappears without medication, because the infection may persist even though no pain is present.

Additional information may be found in the sections on Fever (p. 19), Colds (p. 22), and Swimmer's ear (p. 88).

USING THE TELEPHONE

COMMON COMPLAINTS

MINOR INFECTIONS

INFECTIOUS DISEASES

EMERGENCY PROBLEMS

NEW INFANT CARE

PEDIATRIC PROBLEMS

USING THE
TELEPHONE

COMMON
COMPLAINTS

MINOR
INFECTIONS

INFECTIOUS
DISEASES

EMERGENCY
PROBLEMS

NEW INFANT
CARE

PEDIATRIC
PROBLEMS

COUGH

What the doctor needs to know:

1. *Age:* How old is your child?
2. *Duration:* How long has he been sick?
3. *Timing:* Does the cough occur during the entire day or only at night and in the morning?
4. *Wet or dry:* Is the cough loose and phlegmy or does it have a dry quality? (If the cough has a barking quality, see the section on croup.)
5. *Cold:* Does your child also have a cold?
6. *Fever:* Does your child have fever; if so, how high is it and how long has it been present?
7. *Difficulty breathing:* Is your child wheezing or having difficulty breathing (pulling to get air in and out)?
8. *Pus:* In older children, does the phlegm which is coughed up contain material that looks like pus? (Younger children will not cough up or spit out any material.)
9. *General condition:* Does your child look toxic or especially sick?

Call the doctor immediately if:

1. Your child is wheezing or having difficulty with breathing which has lasted longer than half an hour.
2. He is less than three months of age and has constant rapid breathing or persistent cough (every five–ten minutes).
3. You feel especially nervous about the course of your youngster's illness.
4. The child appears toxic or especially sick. (See pages 12–13, "When to Call the Doctor.")

Call the doctor in the near future if:

1. There is temperature of more than 101°F (38.4°C) for longer than twenty-four hours.

32

2. The cough is present all day long or has a short, dry, sharp quality.
3. Your youngster has had wheezing that has lasted longer than twenty-four hours and which is associated with even mild difficulty breathing.
4. You have an infant less than three months of age who has a cough for more than two days.
5. Your child has had a cold which has lasted more than ten days.

Treatment:

1. If the cough is present mostly in the morning and late at night or if it is associated with a cold, nonprescription decongestant cold medicines may be useful.
2. The head end of your child's bed may be propped up by placing a rolled blanket under the mattress or books under the legs at the head end.
3. A vaporizer is often helpful if the cough is associated with breathing through the mouth.
4. Cough suppressants may be of value if the coughing is preventing sleep.
5. Prescription medicines for wheezing are recommended if this symptom becomes troublesome.

Discussion:

Coughs caused by colds or postnasal drip usually have a wet, phlegmy quality and tend to be worse in the evening or early morning because they result from mucus in the back of the throat. Sleeping in a semi-sitting position and using decongestants to stop the flow of mucus are often helpful for this condition. When your child has coughing that continues through the entire night, you may help him by opening an adult, long-acting cold capsule and mixing a small portion of the beads within the capsule with food at dinnertime. Because the medication will now last for twelve hours instead of the three- or four-hours' relief afforded by most cold medications, the child may not be awakened in the early morning hours.

Bronchitis and pneumonia more often will cause a dry, sharp cough that will usually be present all through the day. (Bronchitis doesn't occur

USING THE TELEPHONE

COMMON COMPLAINTS

MINOR INFECTIONS

INFECTIOUS DISEASES

EMERGENCY PROBLEMS

NEW INFANT CARE

PEDIATRIC PROBLEMS

USING THE TELEPHONE

COMMON COMPLAINTS

MINOR INFECTIONS

INFECTIOUS DISEASES

EMERGENCY PROBLEMS

NEW INFANT CARE

PEDIATRIC PROBLEMS

only at night.) Wheezing or fever that continues for a period of time are also more commonly associated with these illnesses.

Children less than three months of age who have a cough which has persisted for more than twelve hours should be evaluated as soon as is practical because of the possibility of underlying infection within their chests. Most doctors will try to avoid giving cough suppressants that actually stop the coughing. Although suppressants do make the child feel more comfortable, they defeat the purpose of the coughing, which is to bring up mucus which has settled within the chest. Many parents also give cough medicines to their youngsters because they don't like the way the cough sounds, although the child is perfectly comfortable with his illness. As we described in the section on colds, if the cough isn't bothering your youngster, avoid using medication: use it only when necessary to make him feel more comfortable.

In summary, most coughs are caused by colds or a postnasal discharge of mucus. These symptoms can be helped by decongestant medications when the symptoms are bothersome to the child. Coughs of a short, dry quality suggest that there may be an underlying infection and your physician should be called for advice. If your child is having true difficulty with his breathing or if he looks especially ill, your physician should be contacted on an emergency basis.

Additional information may be found in the sections on Fever (p. 19), Colds (p. 22), Wheezing (p. 35), and Croup (p. 38.).

34

WHEEZING
(ASTHMA, ASTHMATIC BRONCHITIS)

What the doctor needs to know:

1. *Age:* How old is your child?
2. *Duration:* How long has the wheezing been present?
3. *History:* Has your child had wheezing or asthma in the past?
4. *Fever:* If your child has fever, how high is it and how long has it been present?
5. *Difficulty Breathing:* Is your child having difficulty breathing (straining or pulling to get air in and out)?
6. *Cold:* Does your child also have a cold?
7. *General Condition:* Does your child appear toxic or especially sick?

Call the doctor immediately if:

1. Your child is less than three months of age and the wheezing has lasted longer than an hour.
2. She is straining or pulling to get air in and out.
3. Your youngster appears toxic or especially sick. (See pages 12–13, "When to Call the Doctor.")

Call the doctor in the near future if:

1. Your child has had wheezing which lasts longer than eight hours even if there is no difficulty with breathing.
2. She has a fever which is higher than 101°F (38.4°C) for more than twenty-four hours.

Treatment:

1. The child should be placed in a sitting or semi-sitting position.
2. A vaporizer should be used if the wheezing is associated with mouth-breathing.
3. Prescription wheezing medicine should be administered if it has been prescribed by your doctor in the past.

35

USING THE TELEPHONE

COMMON COMPLAINTS

MINOR INFECTIONS

INFECTIOUS DISEASES

EMERGENCY PROBLEMS

NEW INFANT CARE

PEDIATRIC PROBLEMS

USING THE TELEPHONE

COMMON COMPLAINTS

MINOR INFECTIONS

INFECTIOUS DISEASES

EMERGENCY PROBLEMS

NEW INFANT CARE

PEDIATRIC PROBLEMS

4. Decongestants should be given if the wheezing is associated with a cold.
5. Liquids (juice, clear soup, or soda) should be offered frequently, especially if the child has been eating or drinking poorly.
6. An air conditioner may be useful for allergic children during the summer months.

Discussion:

If you know that your youngster has asthma or has had frequent bouts of wheezing in the past and medication is present in your home, give it to your child using the dosage last prescribed, and wait at least one half hour to see if the wheezing lessens before calling your physician. The side effects from most medicines for wheezing may include irritability, trembling, and the complaint of rapid heartbeat. Nausea, vomiting, or stomach cramps may also occur. While these side effects are unpleasant, they are not dangerous and are of concern only if they become particularly severe.

If the wheezing is associated with other allergic symptoms, especially itchy eyes, runny nose, and sneezing, antihistamines such as Chlor-Trimeton or Dimetane, which may be purchased without prescription, will sometimes be useful. Some doctors who believe that anthihistamines cause thickening of the mucus recommend that they not be given to children with asthmatic-type wheezing. However, this effect generally does not occur and many youngsters whose wheezing has been started by allergic sneezing and runny nose will find dramatic relief.

Most wheezing tends to begin or worsen at night. This may be the result of objects within the child's room to which she is allergic (feather pillows, dust-containing stuffed animals, wool blankets, or a pet that sleeps on the bed); more often, the increased wheezing may result from changes in humidity or temperature. Air-conditioned bedrooms may help to control these changes as well as to decrease the pollen count.

It is absolutely essential that parents *avoid smoking* near their child if she is wheezing, since the cigarette smoke acts as an irritant and will often make her condition worsen. Rub-on cold medications, or those with a strong odor that are placed in vaporizers, may also act as irritants. Strongly perfumed items such as soaps, shampoos, hair sprays, scented toilet papers, and tissues should also be avoided with allergic youngsters, as these may cause either sneezing or wheezing.

Wheezing that is associated with fever and a cough often indicates the presence of an underlying infection. The great majority of these are caused by viruses that usually do not respond to antibiotics, but your physician should make the decision as to whether these or other medicines are necessary.

(*Note*: Croup may sometimes be mistaken for asthmatic wheezing. When having an attack of croup, the child will usually have a barking cough, hoarse voice and may wheeze both while breathing in and while breathing out. Asthmatic-type wheezing usually occurs only while breathing out. See the section on croup for further information.]

In summary, wheezing while breathing may be caused either by an infection that narrows the small airways leading to the lungs or by an allergy that causes the airways to become swollen. Specific medicines are available to help the wheezing youngster but those which are most effective are available only by prescription. If your child is having extreme difficulty with her breathing or if you believe her to have an underlying infection, your doctor should be contacted as soon as possible.

Additional information may be found in the sections on Fever (p. 19), Colds (p. 22), and Cough (p. 32).

USING THE TELEPHONE

COMMON COMPLAINTS

MINOR INFECTIONS

INFECTIOUS DISEASES

EMERGENCY PROBLEMS

NEW INFANT CARE

PEDIATRIC PROBLEMS

USING THE TELEPHONE

COMMON COMPLAINTS

MINOR INFECTIONS

INFECTIOUS DISEASES

EMERGENCY PROBLEMS

NEW INFANT CARE

PEDIATRIC PROBLEMS

CROUP
(BARKING COUGH)

What the doctor needs to know:

1. *Age:* How old is your child?
2. *Duration:* How long has he had the cough?
3. *Trouble breathing:* Is the barking cough accompanied by pulling or straining to breathe?
4. *Fever:* If your child has fever, how high is it and how long has it been present?
5. *Color:* Does your child have normal color or does his skin appear bluish or dusky, especially at the lips and around the fingertips?
6. *Drooling:* Is your child drooling?
7. *General appearance:* Does your child appear toxic or especially sick?

Call the doctor immediately if:

1. Your child does not respond to steam after ten or fifteen minutes.
2. He appears toxic, has a dusky color, or appears especially ill. (See pages 12–13, "When to call the Doctor.")
3. Your youngster is drooling.

Call the doctor in the near future if:

1. The croupy cough occurs at a time other than the middle of the night.
2. Your child is more than seven years old.
3. You feel especially nervous about his appearance.
4. The barking cough lasts longer than eight hours.

Treatment:

1. Run hot water in the bathtub or in the shower with the doors and windows of the bathroom closed. Allow your child to breathe thick, heavy steam for approximately ten to fifteen minutes.

Youngsters who continue to have difficulty breathing after this treatment should be brought immediately to the hospital emergency room.

2. If the barking cough persists or continues without difficulty in breathing, decongestant cold medicines should be given and your child should be placed in a bed or crib with a vaporizer running close to his bedside. Check the patient at frequent intervals during the night to be certain that the breathing difficulty has not worsened.

Discussion:

Croup is the name given to a deep, barking cough that sounds like a seal's or dog's bark and has a foghorn quality. This has been caused by swelling of the tissues of the upper part of your child's airway, and may occur as the result of an allergy, irritation to the airway, or infection. It often occurs during changes of seasons and almost always worsens at nighttime. While most cases of croup disappear without treatment, the condition of the child at the onset is frightening to most parents and in some situations may be life-threatening to the child.

The presence of the barking cough by itself should not cause alarm. However, if your youngster has true difficulty breathing (straining or pulling to get air in and out) and is wheezing both as he breathes in and as he breathes out, he should be treated at home immediately. (Note: Asthma also causes wheezing, but only as the child exhales.) Steam is a safe and effective treatment in most cases. Instructions for making a steamy bathroom have already been provided, and most children will seem significantly better after ten to fifteen minutes of this treatment. If the croupy cough has continued but the difficulty with breathing has gone away, your child may be returned to his bed with a vaporizer or humidifier running at the bedside to provide additional steam through the rest of the night. If difficulty with breathing has not gotten better after your youngster has been in a room full of steam, he should then be brought immediately to a hospital emergency room for possible further treatment.

Spasmodic croup, one of the common types of croup, will often improve when the child goes out into the night air, especially during cool weather. These children will be almost entirely without symptoms by the time they reach the hospital emergency room and no further treatment will be necessary. If your youngster had a cold or runny nose before the croupy cough began, his symptoms may last through the entire course of the cold (seven-ten days) although they may not be particularly severe.

USING THE TELEPHONE

COMMON COMPLAINTS

MINOR INFECTIONS

INFECTIOUS DISEASES

EMERGENCY PROBLEMS

NEW INFANT CARE

PEDIATRIC PROBLEMS

Decongestants are often useful and frequent use of a vaporizer is most helpful, especially at night.

If the barking cough is associated with a high fever and especially if the child is drooling, immediate medical care is necessary. This condition might be caused by a bacterial infection at the back of the throat that may close off his airway. Croup usually occurs in younger children and when it is seen in youngsters seven and older, it may indicate a more serious infection.

In summary, croup is a barking cough caused by swelling of the upper portion of the airway resulting from an allergic-type reaction, a viral infection, or bacterial infection. It is usually mild and responds to home remedies but on occasion can cause severe illness. Separating the difficulty with which your child is breathing and the presence of the barking cough or noisy breathing is most important. If the cough is not associated with straining to breathe, it is very unlikely to cause any real difficulty for your child.

Additional information may be found in the sections on Wheezing (p. 35) and Cough (p. 32.).

NOSEBLEED
(EPISTAXIS)

What the doctor needs to know:

1. *Age:* How old is your child?
2. *Duration:* How long has the bleeding been going on?
3. *Frequency:* Has your child had other bouts of nosebleed recently?
4. *Timing:* If the nosebleeds occur frequently, what time of the day do they usually occur?
5. *Colds:* Are the nosebleeds usually accompanied by colds?
6. *Injury:* Has your child injured her nose?

Call the doctor immediately if:

Bleeding has lasted longer than thirty minutes.

Call the doctor in the near future if:

Bleeding occurs frequently, especially if it comes from the same nostril.

Treatment:

1. Place your child in a semi-sitting position.
2. Be very reassuring to your youngster to stop her from crying.
3. Press both sides of her nose firmly together with your thumb and forefinger.
4. A vaporizer should be placed at your child's bedside when she goes to sleep that evening.
5. If there is a history of bleeding coming from the same side of the nose on more than a few occasions, arrange for her to be seen by your doctor.

Discussion:

The anxiety which accompanies nosebleeds in many children is important because crying increases the blood supply to her face and worsens the bleeding episode. When nosebleeds occur in the presence of other children, she may feel embarrassed so you should reassure her that most friends will be sympathetic. Nosebleeds are common during the winter months as a result of low humidity, which occurs after heating systems have been turned on. The frequency of bouts of nosebleeds can therefore be decreased by using vaporizers or humidifiers in the child's room. When nosebleeds have been secondary to colds or an allergic runny nose, they may be prevented by using standard decongestant cold medications or antihistamines.

If your child gags and vomits during or after a nosebleed, expect that the material thrown up may contain large amounts of blood. This happens because blood may be swallowed as it slides down the back of the throat instead of coming out the front of the nose.

The amount of blood lost during a nosebleed often appears to be greater than is actually the case. Although the child may soak through two or three washcloths or handkerchiefs, it is unusual for her to lose more than one or two ounces of blood.

42

HEADACHE

What the doctor needs to know:

1. *Age:* How old is your child?
2. *Duration:* How long has the headache been present?
3. *Location:* Is the pain localized to one portion of the head?
4. *Severity:* Is the headache severe enough to make your child stop his usual activity?
5. *Other symptoms:* Does your child have other symptoms, such as vomiting, runny nose, or muscle pains or fever?
6. *Frequency:* Does he get headaches frequently or is this the only episode?
7. *Injury:* Did your child receive a blow to the head during the past 24 hours?
8. *General appearance:* Does your child appear especially ill or toxic?

Call the doctor immediately if:

1. You feel especially nervous about your child's condition.
2. The headache is severe and occurred after a blow to the head.
3. Your youngster appears especially sick or toxic. (See pages 12–13, "When to Call the Doctor.")

Call the doctor in the near future if:

1. He has a headache which is recurrent and interferes with his activity.
2. There are symptoms which make you suspect that he has an underlying illness.

Treatment:

1. Aspirin or acetaminophen may be given to relieve pain or fever.
2. Give decongestants with antihistamines for allergic symptoms or runny nose.

43

USING THE TELEPHONE

COMMON COMPLAINTS

MINOR INFECTIONS

INFECTIOUS DISEASES

EMERGENCY PROBLEMS

NEW INFANT CARE

PEDIATRIC PROBLEMS

3. Arrange for a complete medical evaluation of your child if the headaches have been recurring at frequent intervals.

Discussion:

Most of the headaches children experience result from an acute illness such as a cold or viral infection. Usually the children will have an associated runny nose, sore throat, or fever. Headaches accompanied by acute illnesses most often respond quite well to the administration of aspirin. If, however, your child appears toxic or especially ill, a doctor should be contacted as soon as is practical to make sure that the underlying illness is not especially severe.

Other conditions that can cause headaches that last for significant periods of time or recur at frequent intervals include *sinusitis* or sinus congestion which is suggested by pain above or below the eyes and sometimes by a nasal discharge that may have a pussy appearance (the frontal sinuses above the eyes do not develop in children until the age of six). Sinusitis is most often treated with decongestants, nosedrops, cold medications taken by mouth, and antibiotics prescribed by your physician. *Allergic rhinitis* (hay fever) causes a runny nose and headaches but is often associated with sneezing, red or itchy eyes, and a known history of allergies.

Migraine headaches are usually thought to be present only in adults but they do occur in children as well. The classic migraine headache occurs after a period of stress or tension and is most severe on one side of the head. Usually the pain is relieved after the child falls asleep or vomits. Childhood migraines frequently begin at approximately the age of ten but may not be present with classic symptoms initially. They should be suspected in any youngster who belongs to a family where other close relatives have a history of migraine. In a small percentage of these children the headaches are precipitated by eating foods containing caffeine, chocolate, or nitrites (sausage meats and bacon). Most youngsters find relief from their headaches by taking aspirin. Medications are also available by prescription which may be taken regularly to prevent migraine headaches when patients get them at frequent intervals.

Tension-caused headaches are most often located toward the back of the head and usually occur while the child is under stress instead of after stress, which is more usual with migraine.

Headaches caused by *brain tumors* are most often worse early in the morning and are frequently associated with vomiting that may be accompanied by a slight amount of nausea. Children with these symptoms may then feel better after they have thrown up. Parents should recognize, however, that a brain tumor is one of the *least common* causes of child-

44

hood headaches, though this possibility obviously causes the greatest concern among both parents and doctors. However, it should be considered only when the headache pattern is of the type described above or when other neurologic problems have developed, such as dizziness, clumsiness, fainting spells, trouble with vision, etc.

Eyestrain, which does not usually cause headaches, is mentioned only because it may be responsible for eye pain, especially late in the day, which will sometimes be described by youngsters as a headache.

In summary, headaches in children are usually the result of an acute illness, especially a cold, but there are various other underlying conditions that may be responsible. Brain tumors are one of the least common causes of headaches and should not be considered first. Any headache that is persistent or occurs frequently should be discussed with your physician to determine its cause and treatment.

USING THE TELEPHONE

COMMON COMPLAINTS

MINOR INFECTIONS

INFECTIOUS DISEASES

EMERGENCY PROBLEMS

NEW INFANT CARE

PEDIATRIC PROBLEMS

USING THE
TELEPHONE

COMMON
COMPLAINTS

MINOR
INFECTIONS

INFECTIOUS
DISEASES

EMERGENCY
PROBLEMS

NEW INFANT
CARE

PEDIATRIC
PROBLEMS

STOMACH PAIN IN OLDER CHILDREN

What the doctor needs to know:

1. *Age:* How old is your child?
2. *Duration:* How long has the pain been present?
3. *Location:* Is the pain localized mostly around the bellybutton, in the upper stomach, or in the lower stomach?
4. *Stooling:* Is your child having normal stools or are they hard, loose, or bloody?
5. *Vomiting:* Has your child been vomiting and, if so, how frequently?
6. *Fever:* Does your child have fever and, if so, how high is her temperature and how long has it been present?
7. *Contacts:* Are other members of your family sick?
8. *General condition:* Does your child appear especially sick or toxic?

Call the doctor immediately if:

1. Your child has pain in her lower stomach, regardless of the side, which lasts longer than two hours.
2. She has grossly bloody stools.
3. Your youngster is vomiting material that is green or bile-stained on two or more occasions.
4. She has the appearance of being toxic or especially ill. (See pages 12–13, "When to Call the Doctor.")

Call the doctor in the near future if:

1. Your child has a stomachache that lasts longer than twenty-four hours.
2. She has a fever which is more than 101˚F (38.4˚C) for longer than twenty-four hours.

Treatment:

1. Offer your child clear liquids for eight hours followed by a bland diet that avoids milk and milk products until the symptoms disappear.
2. Apply a heating pad to the stomachs of older children.
3. If medicines are available that relieve cramps, they may be given to older children.

Discussion:

When an older child has an acute stomachache that is especially severe, the concern of most parents is that their child might have appendicitis. Appendicitis may be present when your child has pain in the lower stomach, regardless of the side, for a period of a few hours. Waiting for one or two hours before calling the doctor is useful and it rarely endangers the patient. This will help to screen out those times when your child is having gas pains. Stomachaches caused by illnesses of a nonsurgical nature are likely when other members of the family have a stomachache, vomiting, or diarrhea, or if the pain is mostly localized in the middle of the stomach near the belly button. If your youngster has actual vomiting or diarrhea, most of the time this is caused by a stomach virus or possibly by eating foods that have not agreed with her.

A *clear-liquid diet* which may be useful later includes apple or grape juice, tea with sugar, flat soda (not diet soda), and clear soup.

A sample *bland diet* which may be useful later includes applesauce, banana, rice, toast with jelly, boiled chicken, boiled eggs, boiled potatoes, and cereal without milk. Milk is generally avoided during acute stomach upsets because it may not be digested well by an irritated bowel.

Stomachaches that occur frequently should be discussed with your physician. Recently, it has been recognized that one of the common causes of frequent stomachaches is an *intolerance or allergy to milk*. The milk sugar (lactose) may not be digested properly, and the gas and acid that result then cause stomach cramps. In some children a true allergy to milk proteins will cause stomach cramping and sometimes loose or diarrheal stools. Milk intolerance should be suspected in those youngsters who have a history of early colic, in youngsters with a family history of stomachaches related to milk or milk products, in children with many allergies, or in children who have a close family member who has a diagnosis of spastic colon or who has frequent cramps or diarrhea. These frequent stomachaches are many times misdiagnosed as being related to nervousness when in fact the nervousness may have been caused by the frequent stomachaches. Also, children who have cramps throughout the

USING THE TELEPHONE

COMMON COMPLAINTS

MINOR INFECTIONS

INFECTIOUS DISEASES

EMERGENCY PROBLEMS

NEW INFANT CARE

PEDIATRIC PROBLEMS

47

USING THE TELEPHONE

COMMON COMPLAINTS

MINOR INFECTIONS

INFECTIOUS DISEASES

EMERGENCY PROBLEMS

NEW INFANT CARE

PEDIATRIC PROBLEMS

day may tend to complain most when they are under stress or are in need of attention.

Sophisticated procedures for diagnosing milk intolerance are now being offered at some medical centers, but the best way to detect the illness is by placing your child on a milk-product-free diet for a period of at least one week. Making the association between eating milk or milk products and the development of the stomach cramps may be especially difficult because in some children small amounts of milk may not cause symptoms while large amounts may, and because milk is hidden in many foods not often thought of as containing milk products. Also, the symptoms may not occur until many hours after the food is eaten and they may continue for two to three days later. In addition, the stomachache tends to be worse in the morning and to get better as the day goes on.

The presence of milk intolerance in children with frequent stomachaches is so common that it has become a practice in our office not to order any laboratory tests or X rays for children with these complaints until the parents have tried the milk-elimination diet first. The elimination diet should not be started until foods containing milk have been identified in the home and substitutes for these foods have been purchased so that they can be made available to youngsters during their trial. It should be understood that in sensitive children even small amounts of milk (one taste of ice cream or a cookie containing milk) may be enough to cause symptoms and spoil the elimination test. For that reason, grandparents and babysitters should be given strict instructions as to which foods are allowed when you are not at home. If the child is sent to school or to a friend's house, she should be sent with her own lunch containing foods you know are safe to eat.

Foods that should be avoided, in addition to milk and milk products such as whey, cheese, and cream, are:

1. Baked goods, especially cakes, cookies, breads, hamburger and frankfurter rolls. Whole wheat bread, rye bread, pumpernickel, hard rolls, and pie crust are usually safe. The ingredients of all baked goods should be inspected to be certain that nonfat or powdered milk is not present.

2. Ice cream, which is obviously a milk product; sherbet also usually contains milk. However, Italian or water-type ices are permitted.

3. Fried foods. Many are not acceptable in the diet because they are often dipped in milk prior to frying and seasoned with bread crumbs containing cheese.

4. Sausage meats that have powdered milk added to them. This is true of some hot dogs, pepperoni, and liverwurst. The absence of milk in sausage meats can be assured if only kosher brands are purchased or labels are in place.

48

5. Some brands of margarine contain skim milk; labels must be read carefully. Margarine made entirely from corn oil or other vegetable products is permitted if no whey is present. Butter that contains only milk fat but does not contain the milk protein or milk sugar is permitted. Mayonnaise that is not made from milk is also allowed. Nonmilk-containing dairy products—such as eggs—may also be eaten.

6. Many types of candies. These labels must also be inspected, with milk chocolate being the most common offender. Dark chocolate is allowed.

After placing your child on a nondairy diet for approximately one week, offer her a large quantity of milk-containing products over a short period of time. Give her milk in her cereal, a glass of milk or malted, ice cream, grilled cheese sandwich, and cream sauces throughout the day. If she was reasonably free of stomach pain during the time she was on the diet and then develops cramps, diarrhea, or gas after being given large amounts of milk, she should be suspected of having milk intolerance and the condition should be discussed with your physician. Once the child has learned that the stomach cramps are caused by milk-containing foods, it is usually not necessary to police her diet as she will start to avoid these foods on her own.

There is no question that a milk-free diet is a major inconvenience, but the benefits are well worth the effort. In addition, the majority of children show improvement in their milk-related symptoms as they grow older.

When milk-free diets are used for a prolonged period of time, children should take daily supplements of vitamins containing Vitamin D. Some physicians recommend calcium supplements as well.

There are many other causes of chronic stomach pain, and all children with this symptom should receive a complete physical examination and proper evaluation.

Additional information may be found in the sections on Fever (p. 19), Vomiting (p. 54), and Diarrhea (p. 57).

USING THE TELEPHONE

COMMON COMPLAINTS

MINOR INFECTIONS

INFECTIOUS DISEASES

EMERGENCY PROBLEMS

NEW INFANT CARE

PEDIATRIC PROBLEMS

49

USING THE
TELEPHONE

COMMON
COMPLAINTS

MINOR
INFECTIONS

INFECTIOUS
DISEASES

EMERGENCY
PROBLEMS

NEW INFANT
CARE

PEDIATRIC
PROBLEMS

STOMACH PAIN (INCLUDING COLIC) IN INFANTS

What the doctor needs to know:

1. *Age:* How old is your child?
2. *Fever:* Does he have fever and, if so, how high is it and how long has it been present?
3. *Duration:* How long has your baby had cramps and been crying?
4. *Vomiting:* If your baby has been vomiting, how frequently does it occur and what color is it?
5. *Stooling:* Has your baby had normal stools, or are they hard, watery, or bloody?
6. *Frequency:* Do these episodes of stomach pain occur frequently?
7. *General appearance:* Does the baby appear especially ill or toxic?

Call the doctor immediately if:

1. The baby throws up bile-colored or green fluid.
2. He has bowel movements full of blood (small amounts of blood-streaking on the stool do not represent an emergency).
3. If the child appears toxic or especially sick. (See pages 12–13, "When to Call the Doctor.")

Call the doctor in the near future if:

Cramps continue for more than three hours per day.

Treatment:

1. Initially, offer the baby clear liquids (apple juice mixed half and half with water or weak tea with sugar) with strict avoidance of milk and milk products.
2. Offer fluids in small, frequent amounts.

Discussion:

If your baby appears pale, sweaty, nervous, or extremely ill for more than 1 hour he should be examined at the very earliest possible time. This is also true if your baby is vomiting material that is green-stained, or grossly bloody diarrhea is present. These signs are suggestive of a problem that may require surgery or represents severe illness and should be evaluated by a physician as soon as possible.

Babies who are crying, whether because of teething or from colic or gas pains, look very uncomfortable but do not look terribly sick during these crying episodes. Almost all babies have at least one or two episodes of prolonged crying and may have a red face, drawn-up knees, and show strain during that time. These episodes are often followed by passing of gas, giving the infant the appearance of having had gas pains. If your baby gets these bouts of cramps frequently and they are not improved after you have fed him, cuddled him, or offered him something to suck on, the baby is said to have *colic*. It is frequently referred to as "three-month colic" because it usually improves without treatment at the end of that period. When these cramps occur in the early evening, usually between 7:00 and 11:00 P.M., they are referred to as *"night colic."* While it is not associated with underlying illness, many parents have complained that it is a trick to spoil dinner but has the advantage of providing your family with a built-in form of birth control. The reason there are so many different treatments offered for colic—including chamomile tea, hot water bottles, antispasmodic drops, pacifiers with sugar, and a variety of home brews—is that, in fact, none of these treatments for colic is especially effective. The only treatment that is reasonably successful is holding the baby whenever it is practical and occasionally taking him for a long ride in your car.

Milk intolerance or milk allergy should be suspected when taking the baby off a milk formula and placing him on a formula containing soy protein causes the stomach cramps to disappear. However, as many as 30 percent of milk-allergic infants may also be allergic to soy formula, and a meat-based formula should be tried next. Milk intolerance should be suspected in babies when one of the parents has been diagnosed as hav-

USING THE TELEPHONE

COMMON COMPLAINTS

MINOR INFECTIONS

INFECTIOUS DISEASES

EMERGENCY PROBLEMS

NEW INFANT CARE

PEDIATRIC PROBLEMS

51

USING THE
TELEPHONE

COMMON
COMPLAINTS

MINOR
INFECTIONS

INFECTIOUS
DISEASES

EMERGENCY
PROBLEMS

NEW INFANT
CARE

PEDIATRIC
PROBLEMS

ing a spastic colon or nervous stomach, or if there is known milk allergy in the family.

Breast-feeding mothers should know that fluids containing caffeine (coffee, tea, cola) or caffeine-like substances (chocolate) may cause stomach cramps in the baby if they are eaten in large amounts. If the mothers are eating large quantities of milk products, babies who have an allergy to cow's milk may also develop cramps since the cow's milk protein may cross with the breast milk. It is sometimes useful for the mother to avoid caffeine, caffeinated foods and milk products for a three-day period of time to see whether there is any difference in the babies' symptoms.

Overfeeding the baby may also cause stomach cramps, loose stools, and spitting up. The number of ounces of combined food and milk the baby can usually tolerate at any one feeding can be guessed at by dividing the baby's weight by two. A fourteen-pound baby will therefore average about seven ounces at a feeding and can tolerate approximately six to eight ounces at one time in a combination of food and milk.

Air swallowing by the infant during feeding may also result in colicky symptoms. Infants who suck rapidly may have a tendency to swallow large amounts of air from the area around the nipple whether they are breast- or bottle-fed. For breast-fed infants, these symptoms are treated by making extra allowances for burping and by propping the infant after feedings to allow air which has been swallowed to rise mechanically to the top of the stomach. Bottle-fed infants should periodically be fed using a different-shaped nipple and should be burped more frequently and propped up after feedings. Almost all crying babies will burp when they are picked up since they have swallowed air during the crying episode. These babies will usually have their crying blamed on gas pains when in fact the gas has been caused by the crying.

Constipation should be suspected in infants who have a history of frequent hard stools, which are associated with straining. Streaks of blood on the stool may indicate the presence of a small fissure or tear at the rectum and is not of major medical concern. Stomach pain in these babies usually occurs only at the time of passing the stool.

Having the contents of the stomach rise up out of the stomach (*gastroesophageal reflux*) is present to some degree in all normal babies. Occasionally, however, this constant reflux causes irritation to the esophagus, the tube that carries food from the mouth to the stomach. This irritation may cause colicky-type symptoms in some babies. It has also been suspected of causing frequent bouts of pneumonia, wheezing, and bronchitis when the stomach contents are breathed into the lungs. Treatment consists of keeping the baby in a semi-sitting position when practical and by thickening the feedings with cereal so that the food will physically have a greater chance of remaining in the stomach.

Infections may also cause repeated bouts of crying that give the parents the impression that their baby has colic. These infants should be examined on at least one occasion to rule out ear and other infections that may cause the babies to be very irritable.

In summary, constant bouts of crying and the appearance of stomachaches in small babies are described as colic only when most of the major medical causes of stomachaches have been ruled out by your physician. When the baby has true colic and has constant bouts of crying and irritability, has the appearance of being hungry but won't accept a nipple, and frequently seems to be generally uncomfortable, many parents feel that no one understands the plight in which they find themselves. Parents become irritable because of lack of sleep and nervousness, pressure from other family members, and the constant feeling that maybe they really are doing something wrong. Unfortunately all this happens at a time when they want most to enjoy their newborns, and obviously these symptoms make it very difficult for them to do so.

If your baby has had frequent bouts of colic and your physician has ruled out the most common of the medical causes, don't blame yourself for the baby's condition. Hold the baby only when it is practical to do so, but when necessary, go about your daily routines. Colic usually resolves itself at about three months of age and the majority of the babies go on to do perfectly well afterward.

Additional information may be found in the sections on Fever (p. 19), Vomiting (p. 54), and Diarrhea (p. 57).

USING THE TELEPHONE

COMMON COMPLAINTS

MINOR INFECTIONS

INFECTIOUS DISEASES

EMERGENCY PROBLEMS

NEW INFANT CARE

PEDIATRIC PROBLEMS

USING THE TELEPHONE

COMMON COMPLAINTS

MINOR INFECTIONS

INFECTIOUS DISEASES

EMERGENCY PROBLEMS

NEW INFANT CARE

PEDIATRIC PROBLEMS

VOMITING
(EMESIS)

What the doctor needs to know:

1. *Age:* How old is your child?
2. *Duration:* How long has the vomiting been present and how often has it occurred?
3. *Fever:* Does your child have fever; if so, how high is it and how long has it been present?
4. *Pain:* Does your youngster have cramping in her stomach; if so, does it happen just before she throws up or has it been constant?
5. *Bowel movements:* Does your child have diarrhea or constipation?
6. *Contacts:* Do other family members have vomiting, diarrhea, or fever?
7. *General appearance:* Does your child look toxic or especially sick?

Call the doctor immediately if:

1. Your child is especially sleepy or difficult to arouse, especially if this is associated with high fever.
2. If the vomited material is colored yellow or green on more than one or two occasions.
3. She looks especially toxic or sick. (See pages 12–13, "When to Call The Doctor.")

Call the doctor in the near future if:

Vomiting has lasted longer than twelve hours.

Treatment:

1. Offer your youngster small, frequent amounts of a clear liquid until there has been no vomiting for four to six hours. You may give her a soft, bland diet avoiding milk and milk products.

54

2. Aspirin suppositories may be inserted rectally if your child has fever which causes her discomfort. Rectal suppositories should be used only if your child is unable to retain medicines given by mouth.

Discussion:

Vomiting is a symptom present in a large variety of illnesses ranging from migraine headaches to food poisoning. However, for the great majority of youngsters vomiting is a symptom of a simple viral infection of the intestine and stomach (gastroenteritis).

When your child has a low-grade fever, stomachaches that come and go, a pale or sweaty appearance (but only just before vomiting), diarrheal or loose stools, or if there is a family member who is also vomiting, has diarrhea or fever, it is most likely that the youngster has a simple viral stomach upset. If these symptoms are not present, however, the parent should carefully observe the child for signs of more serious illness.

A high fever might suggest strep throat or ear infection. An especially lethargic or sleepy child may have an underlying infection of the central nervous system. Vomiting green or yellow material having the appearance of bile, and severe stomachaches that don't disappear after vomiting, may be caused by an obstruction in the intestine. For this reason, *persistent* bile-stained vomitus or persisting stomach cramps associated with vomiting should be discussed with your physician as soon as possible.

In cases where a child has a history of frequent past bouts of vomiting, an appointment should be made to examine the child thoroughly and discuss his problem at length, although not on an urgent basis.

Most physicians do not prescribe medicines to control vomiting for small children since these drugs may have unpleasant side effects and more importantly, may mask a more serious underlying illness that would then result in a delay in diagnosis and treatment. Usually vomiting can be controlled by giving clear liquids (apple or grape juice, flat soda, clear soup, jello) in small frequent amounts (one-half fruit-juice-size glass every fifteen to twenty minutes). Only small amounts should be offered because many children will feel thirsty immediately after vomiting, drink down a large glass of liquid, and promptly throw up again. An especially useful clear liquid is made by stirring one teaspoon of sugar into six ounces of a non-diet cola soda. This very sweet drink has the advantage of raising your child's blood sugar even if a portion of it is vomited. Low blood sugar may play a role in continuing the cycle of

USING THE TELEPHONE

COMMON COMPLAINTS

MINOR INFECTIONS

INFECTIOUS DISEASES

EMERGENCY PROBLEMS

NEW INFANT CARE

PEDIATRIC PROBLEMS

55

USING THE TELEPHONE

COMMON COMPLAINTS

MINOR INFECTIONS

INFECTIOUS DISEASES

EMERGENCY PROBLEMS

NEW INFANT CARE

PEDIATRIC PROBLEMS

vomiting since most children are not eating well during this time. For this reason, plain water or diet sodas should not be offered since they contain no calories.

Electrolyte solutions (Pedialyte and Lytren for infants; Gatorade for older children) may also prove useful as clear liquids. They are usually well tolerated during vomiting and have the advantage of replacing potassium and salt that may be lost during vomiting or diarrhea.

Vomiting is the initial symptom of an uncommon condition known as Reye's Syndrome. In Reye's Syndrome there is a swelling of the brain and liver tissues resulting in vomiting, unclear or confused thinking, incoordination, and in the later stages, coma or death. Because this condition has received so much attention in the press during the past few years, it is mentioned here to remind parents that it is one of the *least common* causes of vomiting. It usually occurs during the period when a child is *recovering* from an acute illness, especially chicken pox or influenza. There has been some inconclusive evidence that it may be more common among children who were given aspirin during these illnesses, although not with aspirin substitutes such as acetaminophen.

If your child develops neurological symptoms such as those described above in association with vomiting, call your child's doctor immediately. However, remember that *most* vomiting is caused by simple stomach upset or a viral infection that will respond to a change of diet. Offering clear liquids is usually all that is required to treat the condition, but it is absolutely necessary to contact your physician if the vomiting continues or if other symptoms suggest that other illness is present.

Additional information may be found in the sections on Fever (p. 19), Stomach Pain in Older Children (p. 46), Stomach Pain in Infants (p. 50), and Diarrhea (p. 57.)

DIARRHEA

What the doctor needs to know:

1. *Age:* How old is your child?
2. *Duration:* How long has the diarrhea been present and how frequent are the loose stools?
3. *Blood:* If there is blood in the stool, does it appear only as small streaks or is there heavy bleeding?
4. *Other symptoms:* Does your youngster have other symptoms including fever, vomiting, or stomachache?
5. *Dehydration:* If your child is less than two years of age, does he have signs of falling behind in his body fluids (crying without tears or making small amounts of dark-colored urine)?
6. *Contacts:* Are there other family members who also have signs of upset stomach or fever?
7. *General appearance:* Does your child appear toxic or especially sick?

Call the doctor immediately if:

1. Your child appears toxic or especially sick. (See pages 12–13, "When to Call the Doctor.")
2. He has not passed any urine for more than eight hours.
3. There are large amounts of blood mixed with the stool.
4. Your youngster is vomiting in association with the diarrhea so that he is unable to retain fluids for more than six hours.

Call the doctor in the near future if:

1. There is diarrhea that has lasted longer than three days.
2. Your child has a fever of more than 101˚F (38.4˚C) that has lasted for more than twenty-four hours.
3. He appears to be getting worse after he has been treated.

USING THE
TELEPHONE

COMMON
COMPLAINTS

MINOR
INFECTIONS

INFECTIOUS
DISEASES

EMERGENCY
PROBLEMS

NEW INFANT
CARE

PEDIATRIC
PROBLEMS

Treatment for infants less than one year of age:

1. Offer an electrolyte solution (Pedialyte or Lytren) for twenty-four hours; then, if improving give
2. One-half strength soy formula (ready-to-feed, soy-based infant formula mixed half and half with water) for twenty-four hours; then, if improving
3. Offer full-strength, soy-based infant formula for twenty-four hours; then, if improving
4. Give strained banana, applesauce, or rice cereal with the soy formula if the baby is already taking solids.
5. Milk and milk products should be avoided until bowel movements have been normal for two days.
6. If you have been breast-feeding, the baby should be placed on an electrolyte solution for twenty-four hours while you express milk manually. Breast-feeding should begin on the second day and, whenever possible, small amounts of water should be given between feedings.

Treatment for children older than one year of age:

1. The diet should avoid milk and milk products.
2. Only bland food should be given. Clear liquids should be given in large amounts whenever possible.
3. Medicines that relieve stomach cramps may be useful if this symptom is present.

Discussion:

Diarrhea should be considered a serious problem only if your child is having one diarrheal stool after another, or especially if large amounts of liquid are being lost. All children and grown-ups will occasionally have one or two loose or diarrheal stools for which no treatment is necessary and for which contacting the doctor is unnecessary. Breast-fed babies have stools that are normally runny and have a watery consistency. These babies will usually have a bowel movement with each feeding, and it is not uncommon for the stool to run out of the diaper.

A five-day diet has been outlined as treatment for small babies because it is not uncommon for bowel movements to take five days to return to normal. You may wish to ask your doctor if the diet outlined above has any major differences from the one he would normally prescribe for you. Remember that when your child is taking clear liquids, stools may remain watery during that time because no solid material is being fed him. When your infant is placed on soy-based formula, stools may assume a gray-green, pasty consistency. A diet of this type will correct most simple diarrheal conditions in small babies and older children, but if the symptoms get worse instead of improving, your doctor should be called.

Giving your baby boiled skim milk is one of the older treatments for diarrhea but it is considered dangerous and should be strictly avoided. Skim milk contains as much milk sugar (lactose) as whole milk does. Since this sugar may not be completely digested when your baby is having frequent stools, it can cause the production of gas and acid, which can make the diarrhea worse. Although boiling milk makes the milk protein easier to digest, some of the water in skim milk will evaporate and cause the salt content to rise, possibly making your baby's blood salt level reach dangerously high levels. Small babies will almost always develop a diaper rash when they have diarrhea, and it is wise to protect your baby's bottom with zinc oxide or a similar protective ointment with each diaper change.

The real danger associated with diarrhea is that the baby may lose more fluid than he is drinking. If the baby is pouring out large amounts of fluid rectally or if he is unable to retain fluid by mouth, your doctor should be called. Some streaks of blood or mucus in the stool are only a reflection of irritation to the baby's bowel; but when large amounts of blood are noted, these should be reported to your doctor at once.

It is uncommon for older children to become dehydrated from diarrhea, and for that reason it is not usually associated with serious illness. However, if your older child has persistently high fever or if he looks toxic or especially sick, you should suspect another underlying illness and your doctor should be contacted.

Most pediatricians will not treat diarrhea with medicines, especially in small children. Many of the drugs do not work well and the most effective medicines are opium derivatives, which may mask underlying illness or have undesirable side effects themselves. Kaopectate is a perfectly safe medicine to use and, although it will often increase the bulk of the stool, many parents have complained that it often does little more than color the stool white.

In young children diarrhea may be associated with an ear infection, especially during the winter. If you have a smaller child with diarrhea and a cold or fever that has lasted more than a few days, arrange for an examination by your doctor.

Stools that are green in color have no special significance. They are

USING THE TELEPHONE

COMMON COMPLAINTS

MINOR INFECTIONS

INFECTIOUS DISEASES

EMERGENCY PROBLEMS

NEW INFANT CARE

PEDIATRIC PROBLEMS

USING THE
TELEPHONE

COMMON
COMPLAINTS

MINOR
INFECTIONS

INFECTIOUS
DISEASES

EMERGENCY
PROBLEMS

NEW INFANT
CARE

PEDIATRIC
PROBLEMS

caused when rapid passage of the stool material has not allowed the green color of bile from the liver to be changed to tan or brown.

In summary, most diarrhea in infants and children is caused by a stomach virus that responds to changes in diet without giving medication. Its most common complication in small children and infants is dehydration from the loss of large amounts of fluid that are not adequately replaced. If the early signs of dehydration (which have been described above) are noted, or if your child has other symptoms that suggest more serious illness is present, your doctor should be contacted.

Additional information may be found in the sections on Fever (p. 19), Vomiting (p. 54), Stomach Pain in Older Children (p. 46), and Stomach Pain in Infants (p. 50).

CONSTIPATION

What the doctor needs to know:

1. *Age:* How old is your child?
2. *Frequency:* How frequently does your child have a bowel movement and what is the usual appearance of the stools?
3. *Duration:* How long has constipation been present?
4. *Blood:* Are there streaks of blood on the stool?
5. *Past History:* Does your child have a tendency toward constipation?

Call the doctor immediately if:

Your child has extreme discomfort.

Call the doctor in the near future if:

1. There are streaks of blood on more than one occasion.
2. There is a history of chronic constipation or repeated symptoms.

Treatment for infants:

1. Initially, rectal stimulation with a thermometer or infant-sized glycerine suppository may be used.
2. Add sugar to the baby's formula: ½ teaspoon for every four ounces for a period of at least three days.
3. Add malt sugar extract (Maltsupex) to the milk or formula if there is no change after three days of plain sugar.
4. One to three ounces of prune juice mixed half and half with water may be offered if there is no change.
5. If the baby is chronically constipated, try a soy-based infant formula for at least one week.

USING THE TELEPHONE

COMMON COMPLAINTS

MINOR INFECTIONS

INFECTIOUS DISEASES

EMERGENCY PROBLEMS

NEW INFANT CARE

PEDIATRIC PROBLEMS

Treatment for older children:

1. First, use a prepackaged Fleet enema.
2. Use a mild laxative such as milk of magnesia, slowly decreasing the doses but keeping the stool soft for at least a two-week period.
3. For chronic constipation, use laxatives to keep the stool soft for at least a six-week period.

Discussion:

Most children will occasionally have a hard or constipated stool. This should be considered normal, and no treatment is necessary even though the passage of the stool may cause your youngster to feel uncomfortable. When the constipation occurs at regular intervals, the most frequent mistake made by parents is to give a laxative once or twice and then to repeat the treatment when the constipation occurs again.

The usual pattern of constipation in children eighteen months or older is that these youngsters avoid having a bowel movement because they have been upset about attempts to toilet-train them, they don't have a convenient place to go to the bathroom, their diet has been changed, they have not had enough fluids to drink, or they have been trying to manipulate their parents. The hard stools that follow then cause pain as they try to go to the bathroom and occasionally may tear the rectum. If blood streaks are noticed on the stool, they are most likely caused by a rectal fissure of this type. Because the youngsters are afraid that moving their bowels will again cause them discomfort, they will avoid defecating when they next feel the urge and another hard stool will result to continue the cycle.

If these symptoms have continued for weeks or for months, they can be relieved only by changing your child's habit pattern. This training period may also take weeks or months, so you should not become discouraged if treatment takes longer than you would normally expect. Initially it is necessary to remove the hard impacted stool that is present with an enema or laxative. Then stools must be kept permanently soft, using the smallest amount of laxative necessary to keep them at a consistency only a little harder than runny. Prune juice or stool softeners may be used for some children, but laxatives such as milk of magnesia or Senokot are usually necessary. The dose of the laxative should be decreased slowly every two weeks, but your youngster should be returned to the larger dose of the week before if the smaller dose is not effective.

Other helpful aids for preventing constipation are to allow time for your youngster to go to the bathroom, especially after large meals; make sure that he has taken enough fluids; and temporarily eliminate toilet training when your child has shown a strong resistance. The iron contained in infant formulas may occasionally be responsible for symptoms of constipation but it usually is not. For that reason, an iron-free formula for small babies or a soy-based formula may sometimes be successful. If the symptoms of constipation have been chronic—especially when they have begun during the infancy period before toilet training has started—and if they are not responding to treatment, your physician should be contacted to rule out the possibility that your child's bowel may not be moving contents through it properly.

In summary, constipation in children is usually not a serious condition although it may cause discomfort for your child. Most constipation responds to changes in diet or in the habits surrounding bowel movements. It is necessary to treat chronic constipation using long-term means rather than a single, quick treatment. If symptoms are not responding to simple management, your physician should be contacted for further advice.

USING THE TELEPHONE

COMMON COMPLAINTS

MINOR INFECTIONS

INFECTIOUS DISEASES

EMERGENCY PROBLEMS

NEW INFANT CARE

PEDIATRIC PROBLEMS

USING THE TELEPHONE

COMMON COMPLAINTS

MINOR INFECTIONS

INFECTIOUS DISEASES

EMERGENCY PROBLEMS

NEW INFANT CARE

PEDIATRIC PROBLEMS

PAIN ON URINATION
(DYSURIA)

What the doctor needs to know:

1. *Age:* How old is your child?
2. *Fever:* If your child has fever, how high is it and how long has it been present?
3. *Pain:* Is your child's pain mild or severe; does it occur only occasionally or does it happen every time your child passes urine?
4. *Duration:* How long has the burning been present?
5. *Irritation:* Is there local irritation at the tip of the penis or around the opening of your child's vagina?
6. *Bleeding:* Have you noticed blood in your child's urine?
7. *General appearance:* Does your child appear toxic or especially sick?

Call the doctor immediately if:

1. Your youngster has fever greater than 101˚F (38.4˚C).
2. He appears toxic or especially sick.

Call the doctor in the near future if:

1. Your child is passing urine more frequently than once every two hours.
2. The urine contains noticeable amounts of blood.
3. He has to strain to pass urine.

Treatment:

1. If there is local irritation at the vagina or at the tip of the penis, your youngster's genitalia should be exposed to the air and a protective ointment such as zinc oxide or Desitin should be applied whenever possible. Hydrocortisone-type creams are useful if they are available.
2. Your child should be placed in a bathtub containing lukewarm water and asked to pass urine directly into the water if he was previously unable to urinate because of the pain.

3. A urinalysis and urine culture should be obtained in a laboratory or your doctor's office after the local irritation has been cleared up or in any case where the symptoms have lasted for longer than two days.

Discussion:

A large number of youngsters who have pain when passing urine have this symptom because of local irritation on the penis or vagina. These symptoms disappear quickly after using a cortisone-type ointment. While this irritation may be the cause, it is still wise to have your child's urine checked at a later time to rule out the possibility of underlying urinary tract infection. If there is a lot of irritation, or if the skin is infected around the genitalia, obtaining a urine culture is usually more difficult and is often less reliable.

When the youngster appears toxic or especially sick or has fever associated with pain on urination, this almost always indicates a urinary tract infection. The fever is more likely to be seen when there is an infection of the kidneys (pyelonephritis) than with a simple bladder infection (cystitis).

If your child is straining to pass urine, this may indicate narrowing of the opening of the urethra (the tube which allows urine to pass). This may be caused by local irritation, infection or by an anatomical narrowing. All patients who have this symptom should be carefully evaluated.

Collect a sample of urine before coming to the doctor's office, since it is frequently difficult to get children to urinate into a jar on command. Many parents have complained to us that after they are finished telling their youngster stories about waterfalls, flushing the toilet, allowing the water to run in the sink, and making a variety of noises in an attempt to coax their children to perform, the usual result is that the parent has to go to the bathroom but the child does not. The urine should be collected in a sterile jar which has been boiled with its lid in water to cover for twenty minutes before use. Genitalia should be carefully washed with soap and water and the collected specimen kept in the refrigerator until it is brought to the doctor's office. At the doctor's office a fresh specimen should be attempted and, if successful, the home specimen may be discarded. However, if a fresh office specimen cannot be obtained, the one brought from home may be used and is usually accurate.

In summary, when your child has burning when passing urine, it usually reflects irritation to the genitalia or is secondary to an infection of

USING THE TELEPHONE

COMMON COMPLAINTS

MINOR INFECTIONS

INFECTIOUS DISEASES

EMERGENCY PROBLEMS

NEW INFANT CARE

PEDIATRIC PROBLEMS

USING THE TELEPHONE

COMMON COMPLAINTS

MINOR INFECTIONS

INFECTIOUS DISEASES

EMERGENCY PROBLEMS

NEW INFANT CARE

PEDIATRIC PROBLEMS

the urinary tract. When signs of illness are present, an infection of the kidneys should be suspected even when local treatment is successful. A urinary tract infection can be ruled out only if the urine is examined in the laboratory or doctor's office.

Additional information may be found in the section on Fever (p. 19).

RASHES
(NOT INCLUDING DIAPER RASH)

What the doctor needs to know:

1. *Age:* How old is your child?
2. *Location:* Where is the rash (is it in one place or is it all over)?
3. *Duration:* How long has it been present?
4. *Itching:* Does it itch?
5. *Appearance:* What does the rash look like (hives or bites, oozing or weeping, blisters or small pimples, whiteheads or pus pimples, or does it look like measles); is it coarse or sandpapery?
6. *Other symptoms:* Did other symptoms occur either before or during the rash (fever, cold, sore throat, vomiting, or diarrhea)?
7. *Medications:* Is your youngster taking any medicines or have you been applying anything to the rash?
8. *Contacts:* Are there other family members or friends of your child who have similar rashes?
9. *Child's appearance:* Does your child appear toxic or especially sick?

Call the doctor immediately if:

1. Your youngster has fever that is higher than 101°F (38.4°C), a sore throat, and a red, rough rash that is worse in the groin and under the arms (probably scarlet fever).
2. Your child appears toxic or especially sick. (See pages 12–13, "When to Call the Doctor.")
3. He has extreme discomfort.

Call the doctor in the near future if:

1. The symptoms have not gone away.
2. You are not certain of the cause of the rash.

USING THE TELEPHONE

COMMON COMPLAINTS

MINOR INFECTIONS

INFECTIOUS DISEASES

EMERGENCY PROBLEMS

NEW INFANT CARE

PEDIATRIC PROBLEMS

Treatment:

1. *Itching:* Stop medications, especially antibiotics if they are currently being taken, and give an antihistamine (like Chlor-Trimeton or Dimetane) by mouth, following directions on the bottle.
2. *Weeping sores:* Apply lukewarm water compresses. Adding medicine to the water is not usually necessary.
3. *Bleeding scabs or whiteheads:* Use antibiotic creams (Neosporin, Bacitracin or Neo-Polycin).
4. *Measles-like rashes:* Avoid contact with other children until a diagnosis is made. Treatment is usually not necessary.
5. *Hives or insect bites:* An antihistamine such as Chlor-Trimeton or Dimetane may be given by mouth for itching. A local astringent, such as witch hazel, may be applied to bites. Ice may be used if there is swelling, especially after bee stings. Very occasionally an insect bite may cause an allergic reaction resulting in fainting or difficulty breathing. Give an antihistamine by mouth and rush the patient directly to a doctor or emergency room.
6. *Allergic, itchy skin:* Antihistamines may be given by mouth. The area should be washed thoroughly with warm soapy water to remove the oil or irritant from the skin, especially if poison ivy is suspected. A cortisone-type cream should be applied three or four times a day if you are certain that there is no infection.

Discussion:

Although rashes may be extremely annoying to children, they rarely create an emergency unless the youngster looks especially sick or has other symptoms of underlying infection such as high fever. It is important to contact your doctor, however, to determine if the rash is contagious to others or if simple methods of treatment will relieve your youngster of his symptoms.

Viral rashes should be suspected if your youngster has a rash that occurs over his entire body and that has the appearance of many individual flat or slightly raised reddened areas that do not itch or are only mildly itchy. If another family member has a cold, diarrhea, or vomiting, viruses from the ECHO or Coxsackie group are most likely. If your child has the same rash with high fever, cough, cold, and red eyes, measles is the more likely diagnosis. However, if you have a young child who had three days of high fever and mild cold and who then developed a rash just as the fever disappeared, a viral illness called roseola is the common cause. A generalized viral rash accompanied by a low-grade fever and swollen lymph glands at the back of the neck is most likely to be associated with German measles.

Antibiotics do not alter the course of these illnesses and there is no specific treatment for them other than to give aspirin when the youngster has a fever that's causing him discomfort, or to give antihistamines, which will sometimes relieve the itching. Decongestant medicines may be useful if your child also has a stuffy nose. All of these illnesses are contagious except roseola which usually affects only those under the age of two years.

Scarlet fever (scarletina) should be suspected in your youngster if he has a coarse rash that covers his entire body, but is more pronounced in the groin and underarms. A fever, vomiting, sore throat, and swollen lymph glands in the neck are also indicative of scarlet fever. If this condition is present, your child should receive early medical attention since the illness usually responds quickly to penicillin or other antibiotics. This illness previously had frequent serious complications but has generally had a milder course in recent years. It is not unusual for youngsters to appear relatively healthy and many will not have any fever. Since scarlet fever is caused by certain types of group A streptococcal throat infections, the diagnosis can be confirmed by obtaining a throat culture at your doctor's office.

Impetigo is a localized skin infection which has the appearance of whiteheads, or sometimes of blisters, scabs, or weeping areas. Some areas of impetigo may look much like a burn from a cigarette. Antibiotic creams, which can be purchased without a prescription, may be applied to the skin and will sometimes cure individual sores and make the infection less contagious. However, a spreading infection can be treated only by giving your child antibiotics by mouth or injection. Since this infection is contagious, direct contact with other youngsters should be avoided. It is wise to cut your youngster's fingernails short because many of these sores will have a tendency to itch and scratching may spread the infection. Although many parents believe that impetigo is caused by dirt, this is usually not the case. Impetigo is nothing more than an area of irritated skin (often beginning with a mosquito bite) that has become infected. The old-fashioned treatment of scrubbing the sores and picking off the scabs should be avoided since this may prolong the course of healing.

Hives (urticaria) is an allergic reaction of the skin. They have an appearance similar to insect bites except that the small hole which is usually seen in the center of the bite is absent. If this rash occurs shortly after a new food has been introduced into your child's diet or if your youngster has been taking an antibiotic, these may be suspected as the most likely causes. However, in most instances the cause of the allergic reaction is not so readily found. It is also not uncommon for hives to

USING THE TELEPHONE

COMMON COMPLAINTS

MINOR INFECTIONS

INFECTIOUS DISEASES

EMERGENCY PROBLEMS

NEW INFANT CARE

PEDIATRIC PROBLEMS

69

USING THE TELEPHONE

COMMON COMPLAINTS

MINOR INFECTIONS

INFECTIOUS DISEASES

EMERGENCY PROBLEMS

NEW INFANT CARE

PEDIATRIC PROBLEMS

occur during the time that the child has a viral illness, such as a cold. In these cases, the hives may last through the entire course of the infection. Relief from itching can be obtained by giving your child an antihistamine by mouth and occasionally by applying calamine lotion. They usually will not last longer than one or two days but if they do, or if your child appears sick, be certain to contact your doctor.

Eczema and/or *seborrhea* is an irritation of the skin that almost always itches, has a rough or weeping appearance, and can occur on any body part. It is usually most severe in the creases in front of the elbows, behind the knees, and behind the ears. There may also be a family history of allergies. Treatment of these conditions includes washing your child *infrequently* with soap to avoid drying of the skin and avoiding contact of the skin with wool (including sweaters that the parent may be wearing, blankets, carpets, and upholstery). Application of cortisone-type creams, when no infection is present, and giving antihistamines, such as Chlor-Trimeton or Dimetane, by mouth, may control itching and act as a sedative.

Contact dermatitis is also an allergic reaction of the skin, but this rash occurs when the skin has actually come in contact with an irritating substance (including poison ivy). This usually occurs on exposed areas, causing the skin to become red, irritated, and occasionally blistery or weeping. If you see a straight line of small blisters, the contact dermatitis has usually been caused by poison ivy. You can treat your child by giving antihistamines by mouth to control the itching, applying compresses soaked in lukewarm water to the skin, especially if the skin is weeping or oozing, and applying calamine lotion if small areas have been affected. Cortisone-type creams (like Cortaid and Lanacort) are also effective and can now be purchased without a prescription, but these cortisone creams should never be applied if you suspect that an infection may be present. If your youngster is very uncomfortable or if there is a lot of swelling, especially around the face, your doctor may wish to prescribe cortisone to be taken by mouth or by injection. However, most doctors will not usually give these medicines without examining the child first, to be certain that they are needed.

Heat rash is usually most severe on the chest and upper back but may be present all over the body. It usually looks pimply but the pimples or blisters are pinhead size. The skin may also have a reddened rough appearance. Children will get a heat rash as frequently in the winter as in the summer because of overdressing. It is not uncommon for them also to get a heat rash when they have fever. The treatment consists of placing your youngster in loose-fitting, lightweight cotton clothing; avoiding wool; and powdering the affected areas with talcum powder or cornstarch to help absorb perspiration. More severe heat rashes may respond quickly to the application of nonprescription hydrocortisone cream.

DIAPER RASH

When a rash is localized to the diaper area, the following measures will help to promote healing:

1. Allow the skin to air dry whenever possible. When diapers are changed, the baby's bottom should be left exposed to the air for at least five to ten minutes. If complete air drying is not practical, the baby's shirt should be pinned to the front and the back of the diaper and the sides of the diaper should remain open. This will allow air to come into contact with the skin but most of the urine will still be caught. Do not use disposable diapers with tight bands at the leg or plastic covers over cloth diapers when the baby has a rash. Trapped moisture and urine will prevent healing.
2. When diapers must be used, protective ointments, such as zinc oxide or Desitin, should be used. However, because it is often difficult to remove these from the skin, baby oil may be used for improved cleaning.
3. At regular intervals during the day, sit the baby in a tub or sink which has been filled with lukewarm water to remove traces of urine and stool from the skin.

If the rash has the appearance of a burn, with peeling or weeping skin, it has probably been caused by a yeast called monilia. This yeast tends to grow best in warm, moist places so that allowing the skin to air dry is of special importance. Your physician may wish to prescribe a specific antibiotic cream over the telephone, but many doctors prefer to examine the infant to confirm the diagnosis. If the rash has many whiteheads or pimples, bacterial infection of the diaper area called impetigo should be suspected. You may apply a nonprescription antibiotic ointment (Bacitracin or Neo-Polucin, for instance) to the skin three or four times a day, but if rapid improvement does not occur, contact your doctor early because antibiotics given by mouth or injection may be necessary. Any diaper rash that has not shown improvement or appears to be worsening despite simple treatments should be discussed with your doctor after a period of three to four days.

PEDIATRIC PROBLEMS

NEW INFANT CARE

EMERGENCY PROBLEMS

INFECTIOUS DISEASES

MINOR INFECTIONS

COMMON COMPLAINTS

USING THE TELEPHONE

Chapter III
MANAGING YOUR CHILD'S ILLNESS

Common Concerns About Illness
Prescription and Nonprescription Medications
Understanding Medicines

USING THE TELEPHONE

COMMON COMPLAINTS

MINOR INFECTIONS

INFECTIOUS DISEASES

EMERGENCY PROBLEMS

NEW INFANT CARE

PEDIATRIC PROBLEMS

PEDIATRIC PROBLEMS

NEW INFANT CARE

EMERGENCY PROBLEMS

INFECTIOUS DISEASES

MINOR INFECTIONS

COMMON COMPLAINTS

USING THE TELEPHONE

COMMON CONCERNS ABOUT ILLNESS

Returning Your Child to School After an Illness

Your youngster can return to school when he has had no fever for twenty-four hours, does not have severe symptoms, and *looks well.*

The reason one day without fever has been chosen is that it is common for sick children to have no fever in the morning, only to develop fever later in the day. When he has been free from elevated temperature for at least twenty-four hours, the chances are reasonably good that the illness will not return.

Your child should not be in school if he has an active cough, headache, or diarrhea. These symptoms will prevent him from learning and indicate his active infection is still contagious. His general appearance is often the best guide as to whether or not it is appropriate for your child to return to school. When he is up and around and looks well, there is little reason for him to remain at home.

Taking Your Child Out When He Is Sick

If you know that your child is sick and your plans to go outside are not necessary, don't go. If the outing cannot be postponed and your child is dressed properly, there are few instances where going out will make him worse. As we have discussed in the section on fever, if it is all right to give your child a full bath to lower a high fever, there is no reason why he should not go outside. A worthwhile rule to follow is that you should not take your child anywhere that you would not go if you felt the way he looks.

Allowing Your Child to Play with Other Children When He Is Ill

During the time that your child has a cough or runny nose, he is contagious and may give his cold to other children. However, if he has no fever and appears well, there is no harm in letting him participate in regular play activities. The problem is best resolved by talking to the other child's parents: If they are protective, they may prefer that your child avoid contact with theirs. If they are more fatalistic, they will often not be concerned if the children play together.

75

USING THE TELEPHONE

COMMON COMPLAINTS

MINOR INFECTIONS

INFECTIOUS DISEASES

EMERGENCY PROBLEMS

NEW INFANT CARE

PEDIATRIC PROBLEMS

USING THE TELEPHONE

COMMON COMPLAINTS

MINOR INFECTIONS

INFECTIOUS DISEASES

EMERGENCY PROBLEMS

NEW INFANT CARE

PEDIATRIC PROBLEMS

Separating Colds from Allergies

Sometimes it is truly difficult to separate cold from allergy symptoms. Both colds and allergies cause sneezing, coughing, red eyes, and runny noses.

Fever strongly suggests that the illness is a cold. Itchy eyes and nose that begin in specific situations—such as exposure to flowers or pets—or when there is a family history of allergies should make you suspect this diagnosis. To make the diagnosis more confusing, allergic youngsters may be more likely to get colds because the linings of their noses and throats are chronically irritated from the allergies and may be more likely to become infected. When you are in doubt concerning treatment or diagnosis, call your doctor.

Treating the Child Who Is "Always" Sick

Nursery and school-age children pass colds from one to the other with such frequency that parents have developed a series of "one-liners" as they make their visit to the doctor:

"If there is a cold in this state, Johnny will catch it."
"We have to stop meeting like this."
"Can you sell me one of your exam rooms as a condominium?"

While these jokes are cute, they are really a reflection of the underlying frustration that all of us feel when our young children may be sick for up to one quarter of the year (eight to ten colds lasting seven to ten days each). It is not difficult to understand why these young children get sick so frequently; look at their play- and schoolmates. Invariably their noses are running in much the same way as your child's is.

In recent years, doctors used to remove children's tonsils and adenoids at about age five to decrease the frequency of colds. Miraculously, at age six many of these children showed marked improvement. It is only in the past few years, however, that it was realized that most children improve at this age anyway, without having had surgery.

Vitamins, especially vitamin C, have not been shown in most studies to have a significant effect in decreasing the number of colds that children have (although there may be a decrease in the severity of symptoms). It is most important during this time of frequent colds to stand back and look at your youngster. If you have the feeling that he looks like a well child with a cold, with very few exceptions your observation is correct. If your child truly looks "sickly," check with your doctor to make certain that there is no underlying illness.

The only way for parents to survive this frequent-colds period (ages three to five years) is to simply resign themselves to it. Frequent colds interfere with school, work and babysitting plans, cause nights without sleep, initiate fights with children to take medicine, and generate parental feelings of sympathy, first for the children and later for themselves. You should take comfort in knowing that this cycle is self-limiting and by remembering that despite all of the inconveniences, a cold is simply a cold.

PRESCRIPTION AND NONPRESCRIPTION MEDICATIONS

Despite the common belief that prescription medicines are more effective than those that can be purchased over-the-counter, many commercial preparations have ingredients very similar to those that can only be prescribed by your doctor. This is especially true of medicines that relieve symptoms. In most cases, their proper dosage, purpose, and possible side effects are described on the label. The principal advantage of nonprescription medicines is that your doctor does not have to be contacted before obtaining them, making them instantly available.

The cost of prescription and nonprescription drugs may not be very different because advertising and promotion of popular brands increase their price to a range similar to (or exceeding) that of prescription drugs. Ask your physician if he believes that specific over-the-counter drugs are of value, and which brand names he prefers. It may be to your advantage to keep within your home a fever-reducer, a cold medicine, a cough medicine, and one or two medications that may be applied to the skin. Your pharmacist may also be helpful in assisting you in choosing brand names.

UNDERSTANDING MEDICINES

Much of the confusion about medicine occurs when parents do not understand what medicines can and cannot do in helping their children feel better when they are sick. Parents often ask doctors to give their child "something to knock the cold out of him" or ask "How long is it necessary to give aspirin?"

Most medicines can be divided into three main groups. One group provides *relief of the symptoms* of an illness, such as fever, headache,

77

USING THE TELEPHONE

COMMON COMPLAINTS

MINOR INFECTIONS

INFECTIOUS DISEASES

EMERGENCY PROBLEMS

NEW INFANT CARE

PEDIATRIC PROBLEMS

USING THE TELEPHONE

COMMON COMPLAINTS

MINOR INFECTIONS

INFECTIOUS DISEASES

EMERGENCY PROBLEMS

NEW INFANT CARE

PEDIATRIC PROBLEMS

cramps, diarrhea, cough, running nose, etc. The second major group of medicines, antibiotics, act against the *cause* of the illness, usually germs. The third group of medicines are given to *protect* the body before the illness occurs, such as vaccines.

When the germ is a bacterium, such as the streptococcus that causes strep throat, an antibiotic (which literally means "against life") such as penicillin or erythromycin would be prescribed. Unfortunately, there are few antibiotics which are effective against those illnesses caused by viruses, such as colds, chicken pox, or mumps. Those that are effective have various side effects that may be as severe as the original illness.

Antibiotics should be given to your child for the length of time for which they are prescribed (usually five to ten days) to be certain that the germs are completely destroyed within the body. If the illness does not seem to be improving while antibiotics are being taken, either the medicine was not taken long enough (a minimum of twenty-four–forty-eight hours is needed before any improvement is usually seen); the germ (not the child) may be resistant to the antibiotic; or the illness may have been caused by a virus for which an antibiotic has no effect. Unfortunately, many doctors still prescribe antibiotics for viral illnesses such as colds because they make the patient feel that the visit to the doctor was worthwhile, Also, it takes much more time for the doctor to explain why he is not giving antibiotics to his patient than to write a prescription for them.

Medicines for relieving symptoms should usually be given to your child only when he has symptoms which are annoying to *him*. Do not give medicines to your youngster to relieve symptoms that are annoying only to *you*. If your child has a runny nose, cough, or fever but is eating well and is not bothered by the illness, leave him alone. Many parents can't wait to start giving their children medicines because it makes them feel as if they are being helpful. All of these medicines have potential side effects: cold/allergy medicines cause crankiness or sleepiness; aspirin can cause stomach upset, low blood sugar, or bleeding; and cough medicines can cause nausea. Those medicines that relieve symptoms usually *do not* shorten the course of the illness but are meant only to make your child feel better. If your child was not feeling bad to start, allow him to have the symptoms of the illness rather than to take the chance of developing side effects from unnecessary medicines.

The types of medicines that may be recommended for your youngster when *he* complains of symptoms are:

Decongestants These unstuff your child's nose when he has a cold. Most do not work well when his nose is actively running but may be helpful as the cold shows signs of improving. These medicines may cause irritability and occasionally sleepiness.

78

Antihistamines These are useful in relieving allergic symptoms such as hay fever, hives, and allergic itching. They often cause drowsiness and may make some children cranky.

Antitussives These are medicines that decrease coughing. When a cough is "loose," a decongestant that will stop the drip of mucus down the throat may be more effective than an antitussive cough medicine. Most antitussives—with the exception of those containing a narcotic such as codeine—are of little value. Remember that a cough has the purpose of allowing your child to clear mucus from his chest. Stopping the cough may make him sound better, but it may actually *prolong* the course of his illness.

Expectorants Medicines that are supposed to make mucus easier to cough up are often added to decongestants to treat colds. They have little advantage over other cough and cold medicines and, with few exceptions, are of limited value.

Fever reducers Aspirin and aspirin-substitutes, such as acetaminophen (sold as Tylenol, Tempra, Liquiprin, and Datril), are the best known of this group. As with the other medicines that give symptomatic relief, they should be given to your child if she has a fever which is annoying to her. Because fever frightens many parents, these medicines are often given to children as soon as they feel hot whether or not they feel sick. Despite the common and generally erroneous belief that high fever causes brain damage, aspirin and other similar drugs should be given to your youngster when she has fever that makes her feel uncomfortable. If she has fever but does not look particularly ill, generally no medicine is needed.

Analgesics Pain-reducers are useful for any condition, such as muscle aches or headaches, that causes your child obvious discomfort. Aspirin and acetaminophen are pain-relievers as well as fever-reducers and may be beneficial in helping youngsters through illness.

Antispasmodics These medicines may be useful for stopping bowel cramps. They may have the side effect of causing dry mouth or constipation.

In summary, medicines such as antibiotics which destroy the cause of an infection should be given for the full period of time for which they are prescribed. Most antibiotics are effective only against infections caused by bacteria and are not effective for viral illnesses such as colds.

79

USING THE TELEPHONE

COMMON COMPLAINTS

MINOR INFECTIONS

INFECTIOUS DISEASES

EMERGENCY PROBLEMS

NEW INFANT CARE

PEDIATRIC PROBLEMS

USING THE TELEPHONE

COMMON COMPLAINTS

MINOR INFECTIONS

INFECTIOUS DISEASES

EMERGENCY PROBLEMS

NEW INFANT CARE

PEDIATRIC PROBLEMS

Illnesses caused by viruses and allergies are generally treated with symptomatic-relief medicines that usually may be stopped when the symptoms disappear and should be used only when the symptoms bother the child and not the parent. There are a few exceptions to this rule, such as wheezing medicines for asthmatics and aspirin for arthritis, but they will be explained to you by your doctor.

Chapter IV
MINOR
LOCALIZED
INFECTIONS

Thrush
Canker sores
Cold sores (herpes simplex)
Pink eye (conjunctivitis)
Sty
Swimmer's ear (external otitis)
Head lice (pediculosis)
Pinworm (oxyuriasis)
Vaginal discharge (vaginitis)
Athlete's foot (tinea pedis)

USING THE TELEPHONE

COMMON COMPLAINTS

MINOR INFECTIONS

INFECTIOUS DISEASES

EMERGENCY PROBLEMS

NEW INFANT CARE

PEDIATRIC PROBLEMS

THRUSH

Description:

Thrush is a mouth infection that affects infants and small children, causing white patches to form on the inner surfaces of the cheeks, behind the lips, or on the tongue. It sometimes looks like a coating of milk but cannot be removed when wiped with a clean handkerchief. This infection is caused by a yeast, called candida or monilia, which grows in warm, moist places.

Most infants or children who have thrush will not usually have other symptoms. Occasionally, they will develop a severe diaper rash caused by the same infection as the monilia travels through the digestive tract from the mouth and out in the stool to the diaper area.

Treatment:

If thrush is present, your doctor may wish to prescribe a specific antibiotic solution to apply to the inner part of the mouth, but swabbing the infected area with 1 percent Gentian Violet solution (sold without prescription) four times a day after meals is often equally effective. The Gentian Violet is much messier than antibiotic solutions, however, and many parents do not enjoy seeing their cute baby smile at them with an awful-looking purple mouth. Most bottles of Gentian Violet are marked "not for internal use," but it is perfectly safe when applied in the manner discussed above.

Call the doctor on a nonurgent basis if:

1. You are not certain the infection is really thrush.
2. The infection lasts longer than five days after treatment.

USING THE TELEPHONE

COMMON COMPLAINTS

MINOR INFECTIONS

INFECTIOUS DISEASES

EMERGENCY PROBLEMS

NEW INFANT CARE

PEDIATRIC PROBLEMS

83

USING THE TELEPHONE

COMMON COMPLAINTS

MINOR INFECTIONS

INFECTIOUS DISEASES

EMERGENCY PROBLEMS

NEW INFANT CARE

PEDIATRIC PROBLEMS

CANKER SORES

Description:

Canker sores are ulcers that occur within the mouth, either singly or in large numbers. They are often seen during times of illness or if an inner portion of the mouth has become irritated. Sometimes they run in families and many children will get them frequently. They may be caused by a variety of different agents.

Treatment:

1. Your child should avoid foods that are spicy or salty or contain citric acid (orange, lemon, grapefruit, tomato, etc.) since these foods will burn when they come in contact with mouth ulcers.
2. After eating, the child should rinse his mouth with plain water to remove food particles.
3. Pain-relievers such as aspirin or acetaminophen may be useful. Occasionally you may wish to sedate your youngster with an antihistamine, such as Chlor-Trimeton or Dimetane if the pain becomes especially uncomfortable.
4. Many medicines that can be applied to the ulcers are available in drugstores but most offer very limited relief.

Call the doctor on a non-urgent basis if:

1. You are not certain of the diagnosis.
2. Your child has a fever of more than 101°F, has bleeding gums and many mouth sores, and appears sick. This grouping of symptoms suggests that your child may have a herpes infection of the mouth.

COLD SORES
(HERPES SIMPLEX)

Description:

Cold sores have the appearance of single or multiple blisters that are usually located near the corner of the mouth and occasionally have oozing or scabbing. They are often recurrent and may not disappear for seven to ten days despite treatment. They tend to occur if your child has been sick or has been under psychological or physical stress.

Treatment:

Sores may be treated by applying topical astringents such as alcohol or witch hazel. If a bacterial infection of the sores is suspected, you may apply topical antibiotic ointments such as Neosporin, Bacitracin or Neo-Polycin to make them less contagious. Many medicines are available in drugstores to treat herpes infections, but none of them are particularly successful at it.

Call the doctor on a nonurgent basis if:

1. You are not certain of the diagnosis.
2. The sore lasts longer than seven days.
3. The sore appears to be getting larger or other sores are forming near it.

USING THE TELEPHONE

COMMON COMPLAINTS

MINOR INFECTIONS

INFECTIOUS DISEASES

EMERGENCY PROBLEMS

NEW INFANT CARE

PEDIATRIC PROBLEMS

PINK EYE
(CONJUNCTIVITIS)

Description:

Pink eye is an irritation to the eye which may be caused by an allergy, a bacterial or viral infection, or contact with an irritating substance. The white part of the eye will usually appear red, and a pussy or creamy discharge may come from one or both eyes.

Treatment:

Pink eye that occurs in association with a cold has usually been caused by a virus and can often be treated by wiping away the discharge with a moist cotton ball. If the symptoms are associated with eye itching, sneezing, and allergies, they may be treated with antihistamines that are given by mouth. When the pink eye has lasted for longer than twenty-four hours and a bacterial infection is suspected, your doctor may wish to prescribe antibiotic eyedrops or eye ointment. The drops should be applied to the inner portion of the eye at least three times a day for at least three days, even though the symptoms may go away more quickly. You should wash your hands after putting the medicine in the youngster's eyes to avoid catching the infection yourself. Your child should avoid contact with other children during the time that his eyes are red or have a discharge coming from them since the condition is contagious. It is also a good idea to have your youngster use his own washcloth and towel during this time.

Call the doctor immediately if:

1. There is severe swelling around the eye, especially if it is associated with fever.
2. Your youngster has eye pain.
3. Eye redness occurred following trauma to the eye.

Call the doctor on a nonurgent basis if:

1. You are not certain that your child has pink eye.
2. The symptoms last longer than three days after treatment.
3. The pink eye appears to be getting worse.

STY

Description:

A sty is a red swelling of either the upper or lower lid of the eye. Because it is essentially a pimple of the eyelid, a whitehead may be noticed.

Treatment:

Antibiotic ointments are usually of little value, but in severe cases your doctor may wish to prescribe antibiotics either by injection or by mouth. Most sties will respond to the application of heat with a warm, wet washcloth. Most children won't allow you to apply heat to the skin for any period of time, however, and the minor benefit of treatment is not usually worth the fighting in your home.

Call your doctor on a nonurgent basis if:

1. You are not certain that your child has a sty.
2. Your youngster develops pain or fever.
3. The swelling of the lid is increasing rather than going down.

USING THE TELEPHONE

COMMON COMPLAINTS

MINOR INFECTIONS

INFECTIOUS DISEASES

EMERGENCY PROBLEMS

NEW INFANT CARE

PEDIATRIC PROBLEMS

USING THE TELEPHONE

COMMON COMPLAINTS

MINOR INFECTIONS

INFECTIOUS DISEASES

EMERGENCY PROBLEMS

NEW INFANT CARE

PEDIATRIC PROBLEMS

SWIMMER'S EAR
(EXTERNAL OTITIS)

Description:

Swimmer's ear, which often occurs during the summer months, is a skin infection of the ear canal causing ear pain. You may determine if your child has this condition by pressing on the button (the tragus) in front of your child's ear or by gently pulling on the outer ear. This will result in worsening the pain. Although swimmer's ear causes pain, it does not usually cause fever and is usually not associated with a cold.

Treatment:

1. Your child should avoid swimming or getting water in the ear canal during the time of the infection. If it is necessary to have your youngster's head under water either for bathing, hair washing, or swimming, a cotton plug coated with petroleum jelly (Vaseline, for instance) will usually provide a waterproof seal to keep the water out of the ear canal. Do not use the ear plugs sold in stores since these have ridges on their sides to keep them in place and will make the irritation within the ear canal worse. For youngsters on swimming teams, and others who get frequent bouts of swimmer's ear and must stay in the water at regular intervals, soft plastic ear molds may be purchased at many of the stores that sell hearing aids. These will provide ear protection without damaging the sensitive tissues in the ear canal.
2. Pain-relieving medicines, such as aspirin or acetaminophen, may be given.
3. Heat may be applied by using a heating pad.
4. Eardrops containing vinegar, cortisone, or antibiotics may be used. Most of these are prescription medications and must be obtained through your doctor.

Call the doctor on a nonurgent basis if:

1. You are not certain that your child has swimmer's ear.
2. The pain is getting worse after two days of treatment.
3. Your youngster has fever.
4. An obvious discharge is coming from the ear.

USING THE TELEPHONE

COMMON COMPLAINTS

MINOR INFECTIONS

INFECTIOUS DISEASES

EMERGENCY PROBLEMS

NEW INFANT CARE

PEDIATRIC PROBLEMS

USING THE TELEPHONE

COMMON COMPLAINTS

MINOR INFECTIONS

INFECTIOUS DISEASES

EMERGENCY PROBLEMS

NEW INFANT CARE

PEDIATRIC PROBLEMS

HEAD LICE
(PEDICULOSIS)

Description:

When lice infect the scalp, they cause itching, a rash, and sometimes swollen glands at the back of the neck. Occasionally, the small lice will be noted in the scalp, but more commonly the eggs, known as nits, can be found approximately one-quarter inch from the bottom of the hair shaft. They are most often found at the back of the neck or at the temples. The eggs are white and often have the appearance of dandruff except that when you try to remove them from the hair shaft, they do not wipe off easily. They are erroneously thought to be associated with dirt. Frequent washing or shampooing will not prevent your youngster from catching lice from another infected child.

Contagion:

Head lice are extremely contagious and are usually spread by direct body contact. They can also be spread by wearing hats, mufflers, or coats belonging to a child who is infected.

Treatment:

A single application of a prescription shampoo, such as Kwell, will kill the head lice and most of the eggs. Individual eggs must be removed from the hair with a fine toothcomb or tweezers (nit-picking) since on occasion they may not be killed by the shampoo. Removal can be aided by washing the hair with vinegar and water or with a prescription selenium sulfide shampoo which should be left on the scalp for ten to fifteen minutes. Re-examine your youngster every couple of days for the presence of new eggs, and to determine whether or not he has been reinfected. Linens, towels, and clothing currently in use should be washed, placed in a dryer, or ironed with special attention given to the seams. Usually ironing or placing the laundry in the dryer is all that is necessary to kill the eggs.

90

It is not necessary to treat other family members unless either eggs or lice have been noted in their hair. Some of the medicines used to treat head lice have the potential for causing neurological side effects if used frequently. They will not prevent you from getting the infection.

Call the doctor on a nonurgent basis if:

1. You believe that your child has head lice.
2. Areas of localized infection of the scalp or skin are present. This may sometimes happen if your child has been scratching the affected areas.

USING THE
TELEPHONE

COMMON
COMPLAINTS

MINOR
INFECTIONS

INFECTIOUS
DISEASES

EMERGENCY
PROBLEMS

NEW INFANT
CARE

PEDIATRIC
PROBLEMS

PINWORM
(OXYURIASIS)

Description:

Pinworm, an infection of the rectum and occasionally the vagina, causes extreme itching in these areas, especially late at night or early in the morning. Pinworms are about one-quarter inch long. They are white in color and have the appearance of a thick thread. If infected children are examined late at night or early in the morning, these tiny worms may be noticed.

Contagion:

This infection spreads easily from one person to another since itching causes patients to scratch near their rectum and the tiny, microscopic worm eggs, which are on the fingers, may then be passed to other family members by touching them, or on food or other objects. The tiny worm eggs may also be transferred if you have handled an infected child's underwear, pajamas, or diaper and then not washed your hands before preparing food. The presence of pinworm within a family has no relationship to cleanliness and, although most parents are horrified to learn that their children have been infected by worms, they should not feel guilty about their presence.

Treatment:

Prescription medicines are used for the *entire family* since in most cases more than one family member has been infected. All of the family members should take their medicine at the same time and all linens, towels, and bed clothes should be laundered. Special attention should be paid to underwear and nightclothes already in the hamper. During the next few days, strict hand-washing before eating and after using the toilet is essential.

Examination is needed to confirm the diagnosis if the actual worms have not been seen. Your doctor may wish to place a piece of Scotch tape across your child's rectum and then examine it under microscope to see if tiny worm eggs are present. Many parents make the mistake of washing their child's bottom just before coming to the doctor. This will remove the eggs and may cause a falsely negative test. When your child has constant rectal or vaginal itching, more than one test may be necessary to make an accurate diagnosis.

USING THE TELEPHONE

COMMON COMPLAINTS

MINOR INFECTIONS

INFECTIOUS DISEASES

EMERGENCY PROBLEMS

NEW INFANT CARE

PEDIATRIC PROBLEMS

USING THE TELEPHONE

COMMON COMPLAINTS

MINOR INFECTIONS

INFECTIOUS DISEASES

EMERGENCY PROBLEMS

NEW INFANT CARE

PEDIATRIC PROBLEMS

VAGINAL DISCHARGE
(VAGINITIS)

What the doctor needs to know:

1. *Age:* How old is your child?
2. *Duration:* How long has discharge been present?
3. *Appearance:* Is the discharge clear, creamy, or bloody?
4. *Odor:* Does the discharge have a foul smell or bad odor?
5. *Medicines:* Has your youngster been taking any recent medicines, including antibiotics or hormones?

Description:

A discharge from an infant's vagina may occur during the *first few days of life* since the high hormone levels that were present during the mother's pregnancy crossed to the baby and then caused the baby to have menstrual-type bleeding as these hormone levels fell. This discharge may also have a consistency of thick, mucousy material, which is normal. This discharge is self-limited and no treatment is necessary, although almost all parents feel nervous when it is first noticed.

Vaginal discharge in children between the ages of three and six is most often related to:

1. Not wiping the rectum properly, allowing stool to be wiped up across the vagina.

2. Using bubble bath, which can act as a local irritant.

3. Nylon underwear that does not allow absorption of perspiration and urine.

4. Occasionally a foreign body, such as a hairpin or piece of crayon, may have been placed in the vagina by the youngster and then causes a foul-smelling or bloody discharge.

Vaginal discharge in teenagers who are menstruating is caused by the same agents as those seen in adults. All cases of vaginal discharge in teenagers should be evaluated. However, it is common for early pubertal teenagers to complain of a constant wetness because of a clear odorless discharge caused by their newly increased production of hormones. No treatment is usually necessary for this condition.

Treatment:

1. Sit the youngster in a bathtub of lukewarm water once or twice a day.
2. Have her wear white cotton underpants that are not overly tight.
3. Avoid bubble baths.
4. Wipe the vaginal area front to back, or separately from the rectal area following a bowel movement.

These suggestions are usually all that is necessary for treatment. Your doctor may suggest a trial of a broad-spectrum antibiotic like ampicillin to treat those infections caused by stool entering the vagina, or he may recommend other methods of cleaning the vaginal area such as using a syringe filled with vinegar. Unfortunately, most children will not allow you to use local treatment, and they must be approached using a very gentle manner.

Any persistent vaginal discharge should be carefully evaluated by your doctor.

USING THE
TELEPHONE

COMMON
COMPLAINTS

MINOR
INFECTIONS

INFECTIOUS
DISEASES

EMERGENCY
PROBLEMS

NEW INFANT
CARE

PEDIATRIC
PROBLEMS

ATHLETE'S FOOT
(TINEA PEDIS)

Description:

Athlete's foot is a fungus infection of the area between the toes. It may cause cracking or fissuring of the skin and sometimes results in weeping, redness, or small blisters.

Contagion:

It is technically difficult to spread athlete's foot from one person's foot to another, but it is usually suggested that a person with this infection wear shower slippers when walking in areas that are frequented by other people with bare feet (showers and pools).

Treatment:

1. The feet should be exposed to the air as frequently as possible.
2. Your pharmacist will supply you with nonprescription antifungal medicines that are usually effective.

Call your doctor on a nonurgent basis if:

1. You are not certain that your child has athlete's foot.
2. The rash worsens after two weeks of using nonprescription medicine.
3. Redness or irritation spreads to areas other than between the toes.

Chapter V
INFECTIOUS DISEASES

Scarlet fever (scarletina)
Measles (rubeola)
German measles (rubella)
Roseola (exanthem subitum)
Fifth disease (erythema infectiosum)
Chicken pox (varicella)
Mumps (epidemic parotitis)
Infectious mononucleosis
Hepatitis

USING THE TELEPHONE

COMMON COMPLAINTS

MINOR INFECTIONS

INFECTIOUS DISEASES

EMERGENCY PROBLEMS

NEW INFANT CARE

PEDIATRIC PROBLEMS

USING THE TELEPHONE

COMMON COMPLAINTS

MINOR INFECTIONS

INFECTIOUS DISEASES

EMERGENCY PROBLEMS

NEW INFANT CARE

PEDIATRIC PROBLEMS

SCARLET FEVER
(SCARLETINA)

Description:

Scarlet fever is an illness that usually occurs in children and is caused by group A streptococcus bacterium. It is technically a variant of strep throat.

Youngsters with scarlet fever have a rash over most of the body. It is rough and red and becomes pale for short periods of time when pressed with your fingers. It is worse in the arm creases and the groin. The tongue may also have a red or coated appearance. The rash usually occurs one or two days after the child has developed a fever, sore throat, and swollen glands. Many children initially have some vomiting as well.

In recent years, the symptoms of scarlet fever have been milder than previously, but the illness does have the potential for causing complications in a *small percentage* of these patients. Complications include ear infections, infections of lymph nodes, rheumatic fever, or kidney involvement (acute glomerulonephritis). Generally, the great majority of these children respond quickly to antibiotics such as penicillin or erythromycin.

Contagion:

This illness is spread in much the same way as a cold, through germs passed by coughing and sneezing. Your child should be isolated until you are certain of his diagnosis, and he should be considered contagious until he has been taking antibiotics for at least twenty-four hours.

Treatment:

Initially aspirin can be given if your youngster has fever and is uncomfortable, but antibiotics must be obtained from your physician.

Treatment of contacts:

Contacts should have throat cultures taken and may be started on antibiotics until the results of the culture are known. If the contacts have a positive throat culture, they should then be treated for ten days with antibiotics.

Call the doctor immediately if:

Your child has a rash or a history that suggests scarlet fever. This youngster should be examined as soon as possible, even if the other symptoms are mild. Children with mild illness are just as contagious as those who are more seriously ill and should be watched carefully because of the possibility that they may develop the infrequent complications of this disease.

Additional information may be found in the sections on Fever (p. 19) and Sore Throat (p. 26).

USING THE TELEPHONE

COMMON COMPLAINTS

MINOR INFECTIONS

INFECTIOUS DISEASES

EMERGENCY PROBLEMS

NEW INFANT CARE

PEDIATRIC PROBLEMS

USING THE TELEPHONE

COMMON COMPLAINTS

MINOR INFECTIONS

INFECTIOUS DISEASES

EMERGENCY PROBLEMS

NEW INFANT CARE

PEDIATRIC PROBLEMS

MEASLES
(RUBEOLA)

Description:

Measles is a viral infection that causes a red rash over most of the body, but usually has no or very little itching. The rash often appears blotchy, irregular, and flat or slightly raised. It usually begins on the face and later spreads to the chest, stomach, and arms and legs. The rash will usually appear after three to five days of a cold, cough, red eyes, and fever in the range of 101°–104° F(38.4°–40°C). The duration of the illness is usually about seven days.

Contagion:

Your child is most contagious during the time she has cold symptoms but before the rash breaks out. A youngster suspected of having measles should be kept in isolation for at least four days after the rash develops. Measles is usually spread by sneezing and coughing, in much the same manner as a cold, but the virus is also present in urine. The incubation period is ten-twelve days from the time of exposure.

Treatment:

1. Aspirin may be given if your child has fever resulting in discomfort.
2. Cold preparations may be used for the runny nose and cough if your youngster is bothered by these symptoms.
3. Dark glasses may be worn if the light hurts your child's eyes.

Treatment of contacts:

Children who have been exposed to measles, and who have no past history of having had the illness and haven't been vaccinated against it, should receive an injection of gamma globulin from a doctor. Children who have not been vaccinated and who have received gamma globulin should not receive a vaccination against measles until at least eight weeks have passed, since the gamma globulin may protect them from the vaccine as well as from the illness.

Call the doctor on a nonurgent basis if:

You believe that your child has measles. Always call your physician to confirm the diagnosis. Antibiotics usually do not help this illness but they may be useful for the complications of measles, which include ear infections and pneumonia.

If your child becomes increasingly ill during the time that she has measles—and especially if she develops prolonged episodes of sleeping or vomiting—your physician should be contacted at once. Infection causing inflammation of the brain matter (encephalitis) can occur in one in one thousand infected youngsters.

Discussion:

Because some children who have been immunized develop only partial protection from the measles virus, it has not been uncommon for doctors to see some signs of measles without evidence of the entire grouping of symptoms. Children who have partial immunity may develop a rash with only mild illness, or they may develop a fever, red eyes, and runny nose without a rash. Partially protected teenagers may also develop a rash that has an allergic appearance. All children who were previously immunized with a vaccine they received together with gamma globulin, or those who were immunized before their first birthday, should receive a second booster immunization to insure more complete protection.

Additional information may be found in the sections on Fever (p. 19), Colds (p. 22), and Cough (p. 32).

USING THE TELEPHONE

COMMON COMPLAINTS

MINOR INFECTIONS

INFECTIOUS DISEASES

EMERGENCY PROBLEMS

NEW INFANT CARE

PEDIATRIC PROBLEMS

GERMAN MEASLES
(RUBELLA)

Description:

German measles is a viral infection that causes a rash over the entire body. The rash is red and has individual, flat, or slightly raised areas that begin on the face and later spread to cover the entire body. Most children are not sick before the rash begins and most have no cold symptoms. Usually the fever is less than 101°F (38.4°C), and many youngsters will have chains of tender lymph glands in the back of the neck. The rash usually fades by the third day and most often does not itch.

Contagion:

Your youngster is contagious for seven days before and five days after the rash breaks out. It is usually spread in the same manner as a cold (by coughing, sneezing and kissing), but the virus is also found in urine and stools. The incubation period is two weeks on the average, but can be as long as twenty-one days. Your child should avoid contact with others but especially with pregnant women.

Treatment:

Although no treatment is usually necessary, aspirin may be given for achiness or the discomfort of fever.

Treatment of contacts:

A pregnant woman who has been exposed to a child with German measles should have a blood test performed shortly after exposure. The test should be repeated after two or three weeks to determine whether or not she has developed an active infection. This is important because some individuals may not develop signs of active infection, especially when they have been protected by the German measles vaccine.

A pregnant woman who is exposed to documented German measles should call her physician within 24 hours for advice.

Exposed individuals who are not pregnant require no treatment.

Call the doctor on a nonurgent basis if:

You believe your child has German measles. Many other viruses can cause rashes and illness that look similar to German measles. In fact, it is not uncommon for parents to think their youngster has contracted German measles when in fact she has never had the disease.

Additional information may be found in the sections on Fever (p. 19) and Colds (p. 22).

USING THE
TELEPHONE

COMMON
COMPLAINTS

MINOR
INFECTIONS

INFECTIOUS
DISEASES

EMERGENCY
PROBLEMS

NEW INFANT
CARE

PEDIATRIC
PROBLEMS

USING THE TELEPHONE

COMMON COMPLAINTS

MINOR INFECTIONS

INFECTIOUS DISEASES

EMERGENCY PROBLEMS

NEW INFANT CARE

PEDIATRIC PROBLEMS

ROSEOLA
(EXANTHEM SUBITUM)

Description:

Roseola is a viral illness that usually occurs in children under two years of age. The rash caused by roseola normally does not itch. It covers the entire body and is red, flat, or slightly raised. It often appears worse over the stomach and chest.

Most children with roseola have high fevers of 102°–106°F (39°–41.2°C) for about three days before the rash breaks out. This rash becomes most obvious as the child's temperature falls to normal. It will usually last from one to three days without the fever returning. Many small children will also have symptoms of a cold, swelling of the lymph nodes in the back of the neck, crankiness, and loss of appetite, but others may have almost no symptoms except fever.

Contagion:

Roseola usually does not occur in children over two years of age and it is considered to have a very low degree of contagion. However, it is wise to keep your child away from other young children until the rash completely disappears.

Treatment:

Aspirin and sponging may be used to lower the temperature if your child feels uncomfortable from the fever.

Treatment of contacts:

None.

Call the doctor on a nonurgent basis if:

You are not certain of the diagnosis.

Discussion:

It is not uncommon for roseola to be misdiagnosed as an allergic reaction to antibiotics, especially penicillin, since many youngsters will have had an early cold, high fever, and often the appearance of an ear infection. The child may have been placed on antibiotics by a physician during this early period before the onset of the rash; in its early phases, it is impossible to tell that the illness is roseola. If a patient is taking antibiotics and develops a rash that looks like hives or is especially itchy, this probably represents a true drug allergy. On the other hand, if the rash has the appearance described earlier, it has probably been caused by the virus. In either case, stop antibiotics (if they are being given) when the rash breaks out, and contact your doctor for further advice.

USING THE TELEPHONE

COMMON COMPLAINTS

MINOR INFECTIONS

INFECTIOUS DISEASES

EMERGENCY PROBLEMS

NEW INFANT CARE

PEDIATRIC PROBLEMS

105

USING THE TELEPHONE

COMMON COMPLAINTS

MINOR INFECTIONS

INFECTIOUS DISEASES

EMERGENCY PROBLEMS

NEW INFANT CARE

PEDIATRIC PROBLEMS

FIFTH DISEASE
(ERYTHEMA INFECTIOSUM)

Description:

Fifth disease is a viral illness that causes two distinct rashes. The first is a bright red, slightly raised rash on the cheeks that gives them the appearance of having been slapped. There is also a rash that develops over the rest of the body, which is flat or slightly raised and which has a lacey type of pattern. These rashes usually do not itch and have a tendency to fade and then return over a period of hours. There is usually no fever or other symptom. Most children are not sick before the rash breaks out. The usual course of this illness is ten days, but it may last for as long as five weeks.

Contagion:

While this virus is contagious, affected children are usually not isolated because those who contract fifth disease most often do not become ill from it. They are allowed to attend school and have no restrictions on activity. The incubation period is one to two weeks.

Treatment:

None.

Treatment of contacts:

None.

Call your doctor on a nonurgent basis if:

You are not certain of the diagnosis. This rash can sometimes be confused with scarlet fever.

CHICKEN POX
(VARICELLA)

Description:

Chicken pox causes a rash that has the appearance of blisters on a red base. It is sometimes described as looking like "dew drops on a rose petal." The individual red marks are about the size of an insect bite. The rash begins on the chest and stomach and later spreads to the arms, legs, and face. Children with chicken pox usually have a low-grade fever although it may occasionally be high. The individual sores of chicken pox change from blisters to whiteheads and later to scabs, especially when they have been scratched because of itching. Other symptoms seen with chicken pox depend on the location of the sores. A common complaint is a sore throat, which occurs when the sores are in the mouth.

Contagion:

Your child is considered contagious for one or two days before the rash breaks out and for about one week afterward, but the scabs may last for a longer period of time. The virus is spread in the same manner as a cold but is also found in the individual sores. The incubation period is ten to twenty-one days, but about two weeks is usual.

Treatment:

1. Antihistamines such as Chlor-Trimeton or Dimetane may be given for itching and sedation, if necessary.
2. Aspirin or acetaminophen may be given if your child has fever which causes him discomfort. (Some authorities have recommended that aspirin not be used for children with chicken pox because of a somewhat higher incidence of Reye's Syndrome seen in its use in association with this infection. See the section on vomiting.)
3. Throat lozenges and avoidance of spicy foods or citrus fruits are helpful if sore throat is present.
4. Your youngster should be kept away from other children for a period of about seven days after the rash develops.

107

USING THE TELEPHONE

COMMON COMPLAINTS

MINOR INFECTIONS

INFECTIOUS DISEASES

EMERGENCY PROBLEMS

NEW INFANT CARE

PEDIATRIC PROBLEMS

USING THE
TELEPHONE

COMMON
COMPLAINTS

MINOR
INFECTIONS

INFECTIOUS
DISEASES

EMERGENCY
PROBLEMS

NEW INFANT
CARE

PEDIATRIC
PROBLEMS

Treatment of contacts:

Although no treatment is usually indicated, children who have severe underlying chronic illnesses such as kidney disease or leukemia should immediately contact their physicians to obtain a special form of gamma globulin called zoster immune globulin which may modify or prevent the disease.

Call the doctor immediately if:

Your child has unusual or severe symptoms such as constant vomiting, high fever, prolonged episodes of sleeping, or if he appears especially sick.

Call the doctor in the near future if:

1. You are not certain that your child has chicken pox.
2. The symptoms are not controlled by the treatment that has been described.

Additional information may be found in the section on Fever (p. 19).

MUMPS
(EPIDEMIC PAROTITIS)

Description:

Mumps is a viral illness that causes tender swelling of the glands that make saliva, giving the appearance of swelling in front of one or both ears. Mumps usually lasts for a period of seven to ten days, and often causes ear pain that is made worse by chewing or swallowing. Some children have fevers in the high range, but many have no fever at all.

Contagion:

Your youngster is considered contagious for seven days before the swelling occurs and remains contagious until the swelling has disappeared (usually about one week). The illness is spread in much the same manner as a cold (by coughing, sneezing and kissing). The incubation period is twelve to twenty-four days, with sixteen days being the average.

Treatment:

While usually none is necessary, aspirin or acetaminophen may be given if your child has fever or pain and is uncomfortable. The patient should be isolated during the contagious period.

Treatment of contacts:

1. No treatment is necessary for prepubescent children.
2. Males who are post-pubertal should receive gamma globulin if they have no prior history of mumps and have not had mumps vaccine.

Call the doctor immediately if:

There is sudden onset of vomiting, headache, stiff neck, or extreme drowsiness, severe stomachache, or pain and tenderness in the testicles.

USING THE TELEPHONE

COMMON COMPLAINTS

MINOR INFECTIONS

INFECTIOUS DISEASES

EMERGENCY PROBLEMS

NEW INFANT CARE

PEDIATRIC PROBLEMS

USING THE
TELEPHONE

COMMON
COMPLAINTS

MINOR
INFECTIONS

INFECTIOUS
DISEASES

EMERGENCY
PROBLEMS

NEW INFANT
CARE

PEDIATRIC
PROBLEMS

Call the doctor in the near future if:

You believe your child has mumps.

Discussion:

Swollen glands in the neck caused by a throat infection will often appear similar to mumps. When the swelling has been caused by glands in the neck, it is usually easy to feel the entire line of the jawbone just above the swelling. Children who have mumps will often have swelling over the jawbone line. You may find it necessary to have the doctor make this distinction for you.

Youngsters who have been vaccinated against mumps still have a one-in-twenty chance of contracting the disease, so it should not be ruled out simply because of previous vaccinations. Many individuals who have mumps have no swelling at all and may have only symptoms of a cold. Therefore, if a family member develops a cold about twelve days after exposure to mumps, the possibility of this disease should not be ruled out.

Additional information may be found in the section on Fever (p. 19) and Colds (p. 22).

INFECTIOUS MONONUCLEOSIS

Description:

Infectious mononucleosis is a viral illness that causes a cold, a sore throat, enlarged lymph nodes (glands in the neck, groin and under the arms), and often swelling of the liver and spleen. Symptoms of infectious mononucleosis may not be specific and may include fever, loss of appetite, sleepiness, occasionally yellow jaundice of the skin or a rash that looks like measles. Younger children who develop infectious mononucleosis may have a mild illness no worse than a bad cold and lasting only a few days. Older children and teenagers may have symptoms lasting for a period of many weeks, although the acute illness (fever, sore throat and a cold) usually lasts about seven days.

Contagion:

The illness is spread by coughing and sneezing but is much less contagious than many other viral illnesses such as chicken pox or measles. Brothers, sisters, and other close contacts are not usually infected. It is wise, however, for the infected child to avoid contact with others during the period of the cold symptoms. The incubation period is two to eight weeks.

Treatment:

1. Aspirin or acetaminophen may be given for fever or achiness which causes discomfort to the child.
2. Throat lozenges may be used for throat pain.
3. Activities which can cause injury to the stomach should be avoided, since the spleen is often enlarged and may be ruptured if it receives a strong blow. This enlargement lasts one to six weeks. Children can participate in other activities, but will fatigue easily.

111

USING THE TELEPHONE

COMMON COMPLAINTS

MINOR INFECTIONS

INFECTIOUS DISEASES

EMERGENCY PROBLEMS

NEW INFANT CARE

PEDIATRIC PROBLEMS

USING THE
TELEPHONE

COMMON
COMPLAINTS

MINOR
INFECTIONS

INFECTIOUS
DISEASES

EMERGENCY
PROBLEMS

NEW INFANT
CARE

PEDIATRIC
PROBLEMS

Treatment of contacts:

None.

Call the doctor on a nonurgent basis if:

Your child has symptoms that suggest infectious mononucleosis. All children should be examined since this illness may mimic many others. A quick blood test is available to confirm the diagnosis.

Additional information may be found in the sections on Fever (p. 19), Colds (p. 22), and Sore Throat (p. 26).

HEPATITIS

Description:

Hepatitis is an illness caused by many different viruses that infect the liver, causing it to become swollen. Other symptoms include a yellowing of the skin (jaundice), stomach discomfort, and nonspecific symptoms of illness such as fever, loss of appetite, and tiredness. Liver swelling, with an obstruction to the flow of bile, may also cause dark-colored urine and light-colored stools. In mild cases of hepatitis, no signs or symptoms may be present and the diagnosis must be made by using laboratory tests.

Contagion:

Youngsters should be considered contagious as long as they are having symptoms. The virus may be spread from one person to another if, after going to the toilet and not washing one's hands, one later handles food that is eaten by someone else. But the viral agents have also been shown to be present in the blood and most body secretions including tears, urine, and saliva. The disease can also be contracted by drinking contaminated water or eating fish from contaminated waters. Strict hand washing after using the toilet and before eating are necessary within the household, and separate towels and washcloths are suggested. The incubation period of hepatitis is variable, but it is usually at least three weeks and may be as long as six months before symptoms develop.

Treatment:

No specific treatment is available.

Treatment of contacts:

All people living within the household and anyone who has had intimate contact with the infected person should receive an injec-

USING THE TELEPHONE

COMMON COMPLAINTS

MINOR INFECTIONS

INFECTIOUS DISEASES

EMERGENCY PROBLEMS

NEW INFANT CARE

PEDIATRIC PROBLEMS

113

USING THE
TELEPHONE

COMMON
COMPLAINTS

MINOR
INFECTIONS

INFECTIOUS
DISEASES

EMERGENCY
PROBLEMS

NEW INFANT
CARE

PEDIATRIC
PROBLEMS

tion of gamma globulin from their physician. If the contact with the infected person was casual or occurred only in the schoolroom, no treatment is necessary.

Call the doctor on a nonurgent basis if:

Your child has any of the symptoms that are suggestive of hepatitis.

Discussion

Regardless of the specific viral agent that caused the hepatitis, your physician may wish to administer gamma globulin (serum immune globulin) to individuals who hav·, had close contact with the infected patient. In the past only exposure to infectious hepatitis was treated in this way because this virus was thought to be spread by coming in contact with articles contaminated with the patient's stool or by drinking water or eating shellfish that had become contaminated. It is now known however that serum hepatitis, which was thought to be transmitted primarily in blood and blood products, may also be spread by contact with stool-contaminated articles. Both types of viruses may also be found in other body secretions such as tears and saliva, and infection may be prevented or made less severe by administering gamma globulin.

IF YOUR CHILD HAS BEEN EXPOSED TO:

Chicken Pox

No treatment is necessary. If the exposed child has serious medical problems, such as chronic kidney disease or leukemia, your physician should be contacted immediately so that a special gamma globulin called zoster immune globulin may be administered.

German Measles

No treatment is necessary. Children who have received German measles vaccine have a protection rate of 95 percent, and children who have not received a vaccine usually have only mild symptoms after contracting this disease. The major risk associated with German measles is that pregnant mothers who become infected may have babies with serious deformities, especially if the mother is infected during the first three months of pregnancy.

Head Lice

The child should be examined at three- to four-day intervals for the presence of lice or eggs (nits). If no nits or lice are seen, no treatment is necessary.

Hepatitis

The exposed child should receive a shot of gamma globulin from his physician if the person who had hepatitis lives in the same house or is a close friend. No treatment is necessary if the exposure occurred at school or with a casual friend.

115

USING THE TELEPHONE

COMMON COMPLAINTS

MINOR INFECTIONS

INFECTIOUS DISEASES

EMERGENCY PROBLEMS

NEW INFANT CARE

PEDIATRIC PROBLEMS

Impetigo

No treatment is necessary unless the child who is exposed develops a rash that looks like blisters, whiteheads, or scabs.

Infectious Mononucleosis

No treatment is necessary. This illness has a low degree of contagion and the risk of catching it is relatively small.

Measles

No treatment is necessary if your youngster has previously had measles or has received a vaccination against the disease. If there has been no previous protection, your child should receive an injection of gamma globulin from her physician.

Meningitis

Meningitis may be caused by many different viruses and bacteria. Get in touch with the family of the person with whom your child had contact to determine the causative agent. If your child had close contact and the meningitis is caused by *H. influenzae* or the meningococcus, your doctor may wish to start your youngster on prophylactic antibiotics by mouth.

Mumps

No treatment is necessary if your child has been vaccinated against mumps or has previously had the disease. If the youngster has no previous protection, your physician may wish to give him an injection of gamma globulin.

Pinworm

If your child has had intimate contact with another youngster or adult who has pinworm, call your doctor to have a pinworm preparation prepared from her rectum. Do not bathe your child or wash her rectum before bringing her to the doctor's office as this may remove the worm eggs if they are present. If pinworm eggs are found, all family members should be treated as well.

Pneumonia

Many viruses and bacteria cause pneumonia, but they often will not cause the same illness in each person. Someone who has been exposed to pneumonia may develop a sore throat, cold, or earache instead. Generally, no prophylactic treatment is given.

Scarlet Fever

See Strep Throat (below).

Strep Throat

Strep throat, like scarlet fever, is spread in much the same way as a cold. If the contact was intimate, the exposed child should have a throat culture taken, and be treated if the culture is positive. The youngster who has been exposed and has fever or sore throat may be started on antibiotics by his doctor while waiting for the results of the culture.

Whooping Cough (Pertussis)

If contact has been intimate, many physicians will place exposed individuals on an antibiotic such as erythromycin even if the exposed persons have previously been vaccinated against the disease.

USING THE TELEPHONE

COMMON COMPLAINTS

MINOR INFECTIONS

INFECTIOUS DISEASES

EMERGENCY PROBLEMS

NEW INFANT CARE

PEDIATRIC PROBLEMS

PEDIATRIC PROBLEMS

NEW INFANT CARE

EMERGENCY PROBLEMS

INFECTIOUS DISEASES

MINOR INFECTIONS

COMMON COMPLAINTS

USING THE TELEPHONE

Chapter VI
EMERGENCY
PROBLEMS

USING THE TELEPHONE

COMMON COMPLAINTS

MINOR INFECTIONS

INFECTIOUS DISEASES

EMERGENCY PROBLEMS

NEW INFANT CARE

PEDIATRIC PROBLEMS

119

USING THE TELEPHONE

COMMON COMPLAINTS

MINOR INFECTIONS

INFECTIOUS DISEASES

EMERGENCY PROBLEMS

NEW INFANT CARE

PEDIATRIC PROBLEMS

BASIC PRINCIPLES
OF TREATING INJURIES

1. Protect the injured body part from movement with a splint, sling or pillow until it can be evaluated (see the section on Athletic Injuries).
2. If bleeding is present, press firmly *directly over* that specific area until the bleeding stops.
3. Apply ice or a cold compress to the injured part (if your child is cooperative).
4. Whenever possible, elevate the injured part to decrease swelling.
5. After forty-eight hours, heat may be applied to the injured part to increase its blood supply and promote healing.
6. If you are bringing your youngster to a doctor for evaluation, *always drive slowly and carefully.* Be certain that the car ride to the doctor's office isn't more dangerous to your child than the original injury.

USING THE TELEPHONE

COMMON COMPLAINTS

MINOR INFECTIONS

INFECTIOUS DISEASES

EMERGENCY PROBLEMS

NEW INFANT CARE

PEDIATRIC PROBLEMS

USING THE TELEPHONE

COMMON COMPLAINTS

MINOR INFECTIONS

INFECTIOUS DISEASES

EMERGENCY PROBLEMS

NEW INFANT CARE

PEDIATRIC PROBLEMS

HEAD INJURY

Call the doctor immediately if:

1. Your child has been knocked unconscious.
2. He has vomited more than once or twice.
3. Your youngster is drowsy for longer than one half hour.
4. Your child appears sick or complains of symptoms that are alarming to you such as severe headache, blurred or double vision or dizziness lasting longer than one-half hour.

Discussion:

Because the child might have a *concussion*, parents are frequently advised not to allow their child to fall asleep after he has hit his head and to report to the doctor any vomiting that occurs if the injury is due to a fall. However, it is not uncommon for many children to appear drowsy after the injury or to throw up once or twice as the result of excitement, fear, and crying.

You may allow your youngster to go to sleep after a fall, but it is best if you wake him after half an hour to be certain that he arouses easily. If you find it difficult to awaken your child or if he is constantly vomiting, he should be examined immediately because of the possibility of a concussion.

In most cases, an X ray is not necessary since the general condition of your youngster is a much more reliable guide to the severity of the injury than the presence or absence of a fracture. It is uncommon for a child who appears normal during an examination to develop a problem following a fall, whether a skull fracture is present or not.

Instant swelling over the forehead usually occurs as a result of bleeding under the skin. This is followed by a black and blue mark which will last five to seven days. If a large swelling has occurred, sometimes the youngster will develop black eyes when the blood travels under the skin from the forehead to the area alongside the nose. If your child will allow it, place ice directly over the bump to decrease the swelling.

122

Soft, spongy swelling anywhere over the skull in babies less than six months of age, that lasts longer than twelve hours, is not usual and may be associated with a skull fracture. If the swelling persists, these children should be examined by your doctor even if they are acting perfectly well.

USING THE TELEPHONE

COMMON COMPLAINTS

MINOR INFECTIONS

INFECTIOUS DISEASES

EMERGENCY PROBLEMS

NEW INFANT CARE

PEDIATRIC PROBLEMS

USING THE
TELEPHONE

COMMON
COMPLAINTS

MINOR
INFECTIONS

INFECTIOUS
DISEASES

EMERGENCY
PROBLEMS

NEW INFANT
CARE

PEDIATRIC
PROBLEMS

FALL FROM
A HEIGHT

Call the doctor immediately if:

1. Your child is persistently vomiting or is difficult to arouse.
2. Your child does not move his arms or legs with equal strength and ease on both sides.
3. A tender, localized swelling is noted over an arm, a leg, or other body part.

Discussion:

If none of these signs noted above is present, it is not necessary to contact your doctor immediately. However, if these signs or symptoms develop within the next few hours or if you feel especially nervous following the accident, contact your doctor and discuss your child's condition with him or her. Even if the examination is not justified for medical reasons, most doctors will be willing to see your youngster on an emergency basis because they understand your anxiety.

ATHLETIC INJURIES
(SPRAINS AND STRAINS AND FRACTURES)

Call the doctor immediately if:

1. Your child is in extreme pain.
2. One of the bones or joints is obviously deformed or swollen.

Call the doctor in the near future if:

Your youngster has pain, swelling, or localized tenderness that lasts longer than twenty-four hours.

Treatment:

1. Apply ice to the injured area.
2. Raise the swollen part when possible.
3. Limit the use of the injuried part using a splint or sling.
4. Keep your youngster at rest.

Discussion:

When it is not practical to limit the use of the injured arm or leg because of your child's age, or if he is uncooperative, try to arrange for an early examination. A simple sling may be made for the arm by pinning the shirtsleeve to the body of the shirt both at the elbow and above and below the wrist. A finger may be temporarily splinted by using a piece of folded cardboard and two bandaids. A toe may be splinted by taping it with a bandaid to the next toe. Most simple fractures will develop no further damage if that body part is kept at rest. A twenty-four–hour wait gives you the opportunity to see if the symptoms will disappear.

USING THE TELEPHONE

COMMON COMPLAINTS

MINOR INFECTIONS

INFECTIOUS DISEASES

EMERGENCY PROBLEMS

NEW INFANT CARE

PEDIATRIC PROBLEMS

USING THE
TELEPHONE

COMMON
COMPLAINTS

MINOR
INFECTIONS

INFECTIOUS
DISEASES

EMERGENCY
PROBLEMS

NEW INFANT
CARE

PEDIATRIC
PROBLEMS

INJURY TO THE NOSE

Call the doctor immediately if:

1. Your youngster is in extreme pain.
2. The nose is obviously swollen and crooked.
3. There is bleeding from the nose lasting longer than twenty minutes.

Treatment:

1. Stop the bleeding by gently pressing both sides of the nose together while your child is either sitting or semi-reclining.
2. Apply ice or a cold compress to the swelling once the bleeding has stopped.

Discussion:

It is especially important to try to stop your youngster from crying, since excitement and exercise will increase the blood supply to his face and make the bleeding worse. You should talk to him in a calm, relaxed manner to relieve his feelings of fear. Since the nose of a child prior to the age of two or three is primarily composed of cartilage, X ray films are not usually necessary for younger children. In most cases, immediate attention is not mandatory since many ear, nose, and throat doctors prefer to correct fractures of the nose only after some or all of the swelling has disappeared.

CUTS
(LACERATIONS)

Call the doctor immediately if:

1. Your child has a gaping cut which is longer than one-quarter inch.
2. You are unable to stop the bleeding after 20 minutes.

Treatment:

1. Apply pressure directly over the cut until the bleeding stops.
2. Wash the cut thoroughly with soap and warm water if it is small and does not have to be examined.
3. Cover the cut with a clean dressing.

Discussion:

Any cuts on the head, face, or mouth may cause a tremendous amount of bleeding even when they are very small. It is generally worthwhile to attempt to stop the bleeding by pressing directly on the bandage covering the injured area for five to ten minutes. Properly evaluating the size of a small cut will often help to avoid an unnecessary frantic trip to the emergency room of your local hospital.

Unless a cut inside the mouth is large and gaping, stitches are not usually necessary since this area heals quickly. Closing it with stitches may trap germs within the cut and can cause an infection.

USING THE TELEPHONE

COMMON COMPLAINTS

MINOR INFECTIONS

INFECTIOUS DISEASES

EMERGENCY PROBLEMS

NEW INFANT CARE

PEDIATRIC PROBLEMS

USING THE
TELEPHONE

COMMON
COMPLAINTS

MINOR
INFECTIONS

INFECTIOUS
DISEASES

EMERGENCY
PROBLEMS

NEW INFANT
CARE

PEDIATRIC
PROBLEMS

PUNCTURE WOUNDS

Call the doctor immediately if:

The wound is larger than one-quarter inch across.

Treatment:

1. If bleeding is present, press a clean towel, washcloth, or hand-kerchief directly over the wound until the bleeding stops.
2. Wash the wound well with hot soapy water.
3. Cover it with a clean dressing.
4. Contact your physician about obtaining a tetanus toxoid immunization if more than five years have elapsed since the last booster shot. (Many physicians allow ten years before giving a tetanus booster.)

Call the doctor in the near future if:

An area of tender redness develops around the wound and appears to be increasing in size one to two days later. This may indicate that the wound is becoming infected.

ANIMAL BITES

USING THE TELEPHONE

COMMON COMPLAINTS

MINOR INFECTIONS

INFECTIOUS DISEASES

EMERGENCY PROBLEMS

NEW INFANT CARE

PEDIATRIC PROBLEMS

Call the doctor immediately if:

1. The bite results in a cut larger than one quarter inch in length.
2. There is bleeding that is difficult to stop.
3. The bite did not occur while playing with or teasing the animal, especially if the animal was a bat, skunk, raccoon, fox, monkey, or dog.

Call the doctor in the near future if:

1. The redness or pain at the site of the bite is worsening rather than improving.
2. Your child has not received a tetanus immunization during the past five years (although many physicians wait ten years before giving a booster immunization).
3. She was bitten by an apparently healthy or friendly dog or cat that is not known to be immunized against rabies or cannot be located.
4. The animal bite appears to be minor but you cannot get an accurate description of the incident from your youngster.

Treatment:

1. Wash the bite immediately with large amounts of warm soapy water.
2. Apply pressure directly to the bite to stop bleeding.
3. Apply ice over the injury to reduce pain and swelling.
4. Notify your local police if the animal does not belong to your family, if only to make a record to be kept on file in case the animal bites someone else.

Discussion:

Animal bites pose two major problems: The first is to be sure that the wound itself is cared for properly. The second is to determine whether your child is at risk of developing rabies.

129

USING THE
TELEPHONE

COMMON
COMPLAINTS

MINOR
INFECTIONS

INFECTIOUS
DISEASES

EMERGENCY
PROBLEMS

NEW INFANT
CARE

PEDIATRIC
PROBLEMS

If the bite occurred while your child was playing with, teasing, or feeding an animal that appeared well—especially if the animal has been immunized against rabies—the chance of her contracting rabies from that animal is truly minimal. It is also uncommon for bites from mice, rats and squirrels to be dangerous. When you are not certain whether rabies has been reported in your immediate area, this information can be obtained by contacting your doctor or the local board of health. Although it is often a difficult problem for neighbors, parents should contact the local police when their child is bitten by a dog that is not their own family pet. If medical complications result from the bite, the owners of that pet may be liable for those complications, but more importantly, if the animal becomes ill or has been biting other people in the neighborhood, the police report will make it more likely that the animal will be followed properly. If you feel uncomfortable about reporting a neighbor's pet, tell the neighbor that it is being reported at the request of your physician and let the police know that you are not pressing charges but merely wish that the report be filed for possible future use. Whenever it is difficult to get an accurate history from your child concerning the circumstances of the bite, or if you are not absolutely certain that the wound looks clean, contact your physician for further advice.

HUMAN BITES

Call the doctor immediately if:

1. A cut longer than one quarter inch occurs.
2. There is persistent pain or bleeding.

Call the doctor in the near future if:

1. At the site of the wound there is redness or pain that is increasing rather than decreasing in intensity.
2. Your child has not had tetanus immunization within five years (although some physicians wait ten years before giving a tetanus booster).

Treatment:

1. Wash the wound vigorously with warm soapy water.
2. Apply pressure directly over the cut to stop bleeding.
3. Place ice over the cut to reduce swelling.

Discussion:

Most human bites do not have medical complications. However, because they are usually a type of puncture wound, there is a possibility that they may later become infected. In most cases, washing the wound thoroughly with hot soapy water is all that is necessary to prevent infection, but some physicians prefer to prescribe antibiotics for their patients if the cut is especially deep.

USING THE TELEPHONE

COMMON COMPLAINTS

MINOR INFECTIONS

INFECTIOUS DISEASES

EMERGENCY PROBLEMS

NEW INFANT CARE

PEDIATRIC PROBLEMS

131

USING THE TELEPHONE

COMMON COMPLAINTS

MINOR INFECTIONS

INFECTIOUS DISEASES

EMERGENCY PROBLEMS

NEW INFANT CARE

PEDIATRIC PROBLEMS

BURNS

Call the doctor immediately if:

There is any burned area larger than three inches across.

Treatment:

1. Apply cool wet compresses.
2. Ten to fifteen minutes later, wash the burn with lukewarm soapy water.
3. Cover the burn with a clean dressing (a clean handkerchief or cloth).
4. Give your child pain-relieving medicine such as aspirin or acetaminophen if it is necessary.

Discussion:

All large burns should be examined, cleaned, and dressed immediately. This also may be necessary for smaller burns in areas that are difficult to keep clean, such as the hands of small children. Apply cool water to the burn immediately because the skin may continue to cook for a short period of time after the heat source is removed. Many doctors suggest applying antibiotic creams to small burns to prevent infection.

When large areas are burned, some doctors will start their patients on antibiotics by injection or by mouth to prevent a streptococcal infection. The majority of burns respond well to local treatment, but if you believe that healing is slow or if you are not certain about the child's condition, your physician should be contacted at once.

INJURY TO THE EYE

Call the doctor immediately if:

1. The eye is constantly red or tearing.
2. There is pain which lasts longer than one half hour.
3. The pupils are different sizes.
4. A puncture wound or cut is noticeable.

Immediate treatment:

1. Apply ice or a cold-water compress to the outer eyelid to decrease pain and swelling.
2. Acetaminophen or aspirin may be given by mouth for pain relief.

USING THE TELEPHONE

COMMON COMPLAINTS

MINOR INFECTIONS

INFECTIOUS DISEASES

EMERGENCY PROBLEMS

NEW INFANT CARE

PEDIATRIC PROBLEMS

133

USING THE TELEPHONE

COMMON COMPLAINTS

MINOR INFECTIONS

INFECTIOUS DISEASES

EMERGENCY PROBLEMS

NEW INFANT CARE

PEDIATRIC PROBLEMS

SWALLOWING OF SOLID OBJECTS

Call the doctor immediately if:

1. Your child has a cough that lasts longer than ten minutes.
2. Your child is wheezing.
3. Your youngster has a stomachache.
4. Your child has vomiting.
5. Bloody stools are present.
6. The swallowed object has sharp or pointed edges.

Discussion:

Most objects swallowed by youngsters do not cause harm. If the swallowed object is small enough to pass easily into the stomach, it is usually small enough also to pass through the rectum. Coins, marbles and buttons are the rounded objects that are most frequently swallowed.

It is usually not necessary to examine your child's bowel movement to determine whether the object has passed, since it will probably not cause a problem and because in many instances it was not actually swallowed. Taking an X ray of the stomach is also not necessary for these reasons, especially since many of the objects that are swallowed do not show up on the X-ray film. If the object that was swallowed has sharp or pointed edges (for example an open safety pin) an X-ray film may be taken so that your physician can monitor its progress through your child's bowel. X-ray film may also be ordered if your youngster develops symptoms of pain, vomiting, or bloody bowel movements. Most plastic objects will not be visible to X rays and glass objects will appear on the X-ray film only if the glass contains lead. When you are not certain whether or not the object swallowed may be dangerous to your child, contact your physician.

POISONING

What the doctor needs to know:

Solid medicines (pills):
1. Name of the medicine.
2. How many pills were taken.
3. How long ago were they swallowed.
4. If it is a prescription drug:
   (a) The name and recommended dose of the drug, as it appears on the label.
   (b) The pharmacy's name and telephone number.
   (c) The number of the prescription.
   (d) The approximate number of pills left in the bottle.
5. If the medicine is a nonprescription drug, read to the doctor the contents and the ingredients of the medicine.
6. Tell your doctor if your child has any symptoms such as sleepiness, vomiting, stomachache, or problems with breathing.
7. Give the doctor your telephone number.

Liquid Substances:
1. The name of the substance.
2. The amount taken.
3. The length of time since the substance was swallowed.
4. Read the contents from the label if possible.
5. Does the liquid smell like a solvent (cleaning fluid, gasoline, turpentine, etc.)?
6. Give the doctor your telephone number.

Call the doctor immediately if:

1. You know that the substance taken can cause sleepiness or can depress breathing. Examples include tranquilizers and sleeping pills.
2. Your child has swallowed any liquid that has a burning effect regardless of the amount taken. Examples include drain cleaners, lye, and oven cleaners.
3. Your youngster has symptoms of any kind following the ingestion of the substance.

USING THE TELEPHONE

COMMON COMPLAINTS

MINOR INFECTIONS

INFECTIOUS DISEASES

EMERGENCY PROBLEMS

NEW INFANT CARE

PEDIATRIC PROBLEMS

USING THE TELEPHONE

COMMON COMPLAINTS

MINOR INFECTIONS

INFECTIOUS DISEASES

EMERGENCY PROBLEMS

NEW INFANT CARE

PEDIATRIC PROBLEMS

Further instructions:

If it is necessary to contact the doctor immediately and your physician cannot be reached within five minutes from the time the substance was swallowed and he is not in his office, bring your child immediately to the nearest hospital emergency room. If your community has a poison control number, that number might be called instead of calling your physician. However, if you have a strong suspicion that the material swallowed might be dangerous to your child, bringing him to an emergency facility for immediate treatment is absolutely necessary.

Treatment:

If a small amount of medicine has been taken—for example one pill or tablet—or if the swallowed substance is probably not harmful, such as vitamins without iron, you may wish to have your child vomit back that substance at home in order to avoid having it absorbed from his stomach.

If the swallowed material is a solvent and smells like cleaning fluid, gasoline, or turpentine, *never induce vomiting* because if your child breathes in the material, it can cause a severe pneumonia.

Immediately after your child has swallowed the substance or while you are in the car, give your child large amounts of liquid to drink (milk is especially good for this purpose). When syrup of ipecac is not available in your home, take your child to a pharmacy, bringing a tablespoon with you so that medication may be given at the pharmacy without losing valuable time. If after giving your child one tablespoon of syrup of ipecac at the pharmacy, he has not vomited after twenty minutes, give him one-half tablespoon as a second dose at that time. Continue to offer him large amounts to drink until vomiting occurs.

If solvent-containing substances have been taken and your child appears well, giving him large amounts of fluid to drink is usually all that is necessary to dilute the material in his stomach. On occasion, signs of bronchitis or pneumonia may occur one to two days later, therefore, if a cough, wheezing, or difficulty in breathing occurs at a later time, you should be aware that these symptoms may have been caused by swallowing those solvent materials. If the symptoms become severe, bring your child to the doctor.

136

Discussion:

When you are not certain of the number of tablets taken, how much liquid was swallowed, or whether the material swallowed might be dangerous to your child, contact your physician or your local poison control facility immediately. Taking a single tablet of any adult medicine may cause the results for which the medicine was intended (a tranquilizer may make your child sleepy or high blood pressure medicine may lower his blood pressure somewhat), but it is very uncommon for a single tablet of any medicine to cause side effects that would actually be dangerous. If you are not certain how many tablets were taken it may be useful to have the child vomit after taking the pills. This also teaches your child how serious taking medicines without approval might be. Remember, however, that inducing vomiting when your child has taken solvent-like substances should never be done because of the risk that it may lead to pneumonia at a later time.

The telephone number of your nearest poison control center can usually be obtained from your telephone directory or your local hospital emergency room. These centers usually provide twenty-four-hour emergency service. The information that they need has been outlined in the first part of this section, but it is most important to have the container of the medicine or material swallowed in front of you at time of the telephone call.

A list of the most commonly swallowed medicines is provided below:

1. *Aspirin* (acetylsalicylic acid): Aspirin may be toxic if more than one tablet for every two pounds of body weight is taken. For example, if your child has swallowed fifteen tablets and weighs twenty-five to thirty pounds, you should be concerned that the amount swallowed might be dangerous. The initial sign of aspirin poisoning is rapid breathing. This should be watched for whenever aspirin ingestion is suspected.

2. *Fever reducers* (acetaminophen, including Liquiprin, Tylenol, Datril, and Tempra): A toxic dose of this medicine is approximately 65 milligrams for every two pounds of body weight. Symptoms except vomiting usually do not appear immediately after swallowing the medicine, but may occur as long as two to three days later. These symptoms include changes in central nervous system function (such as drowsiness, confusion, or change in personality) or signs of the liver not functioning properly. Jaundice, however, is not usually seen.

USING THE TELEPHONE

COMMON COMPLAINTS

MINOR INFECTIONS

INFECTIOUS DISEASES

EMERGENCY PROBLEMS

NEW INFANT CARE

PEDIATRIC PROBLEMS

137

USING THE
TELEPHONE

COMMON
COMPLAINTS

MINOR
INFECTIONS

INFECTIOUS
DISEASES

EMERGENCY
PROBLEMS

NEW INFANT
CARE

PEDIATRIC
PROBLEMS

3. *Cold preparations*: These medicines usually are not dangerous unless taken in very large amounts. They may cause symptoms of nervousness, irritability, or drowsiness. On occasion, they may also cause high blood pressure. Usually treatment is not necessary.

4. *Vitamins*: Large amounts of vitamins are not toxic when taken as a single large dose, but they can be extremely dangerous if they contain *iron*. X-ray films of the stomach will often confirm the number of tablets taken because the iron within the tablets can be seen on the film. Iron intoxication may cause a sudden onset of extreme illness, possibly including shock. If your child has swallowed more than three or four tablets containing iron, your physician should be contacted immediately.

5. *Birth control pills*: This medicine is not dangerous if only a few tablets have been swallowed. Girls will occasionally have vaginal bleeding one or two days after the pills are taken, but this bleeding is not dangerous and disappears without treatment.

6. *Tranquilizers*: Swallowing a single tablet may cause sleepiness or occasionally irritability. Treatment is usually not necessary. However, if there is any question as to the number of tablets swallowed, your child should be induced to vomit as soon as possible and your physician should be contacted immediately.

SEIZURES OR CONVULSIONS
(INCLUDING FEVER CONVULSIONS)

Call the doctor immediately:

If you believe your child is having convulsions or seizures.

Treatment:

1. Place the child on the floor next to the telephone so that he can be observed while help is being called.
2. Call the police, an ambulance, or a neighbor (whoever will respond first) to provide transportation to a treatment facility.

Discussion:

With very few exceptions, holding the breath, which may occur during a convulsion or seizure, stops by itself, although occasionally the child may look blue for a short period of time.

The patient should be placed on the floor next to the telephone to prevent his falling from the table, bed, or chair while help is being summoned. Because little emergency equipment is usually necessary to treat a seizure, rapid transportation to the doctor's office or hospital has the highest priority. Unless it is absolutely necessary, do not try to drive your child to another location during a seizure because it is virtually impossible to concentrate on safe driving skills. Studies performed on children following convulsions or seizures have determined that unless an infection of the nervous system (meningitis or encephalitis) is present or unless neurologic impairment was noted before the seizure, brain damage resulting from the seizure rarely occurs when the convulsions were caused by fever. In studies where large numbers of children who experienced fever convulsions were compared to their brothers and sisters, no significant differences in intelligence, learning ability, or neurologic examinations were noted.

There are too many potential causes of convulsions or seizures to mention all of them in this section, but they may be discussed with your physician after emergency treatment has been given to your youngster.

139

USING THE TELEPHONE

COMMON COMPLAINTS

MINOR INFECTIONS

INFECTIOUS DISEASES

EMERGENCY PROBLEMS

NEW INFANT CARE

PEDIATRIC PROBLEMS

PEDIATRIC
PROBLEMS

NEW INFANT
CARE

EMERGENCY
PROBLEMS

INFECTIOUS
DISEASES

MINOR
INFECTIONS

COMMON
COMPLAINTS

USING THE
TELEPHONE

Chapter VII
THE CARE OF
NEW INFANTS

Newborn infant care
Understanding your feelings
How to prepare older children for the new baby
Breast vs. bottle feeding
Breast-feeding
Formula-feeding
Feeding schedules
Solid foods
Weaning your infant from the breast
Care of the umbilicus (belly button)
Bathing
Care of the skin
Bowel movements
Taking the baby out
Visitors during the baby's infancy
Smoking near the baby
Traveling with the baby
Watching your baby grow
Immunizations
Common concerns regarding newborns

USING THE TELEPHONE

COMMON COMPLAINTS

MINOR INFECTIONS

INFECTIOUS DISEASES

EMERGENCY PROBLEMS

NEW INFANT CARE

PEDIATRIC PROBLEMS

PEDIATRIC PROBLEMS

NEW INFANT CARE

EMERGENCY PROBLEMS

INFECTIOUS DISEASES

MINOR INFECTIONS

COMMON COMPLAINTS

USING THE TELEPHONE

NEWBORN INFANT CARE

For many years, doctors, nurses, and grandparents have treated the care of new infants as if it were a mystical experience. Elaborate rules were established regarding the sterilization of formulas, feeding schedule protocols, and proper skin care. Rules were also created concerning all sorts of subjects including when to allow visitors to see the baby, when to take the baby out, and how to hold her for feeding. Because most parents want to provide their newly born children with the best environment as they enter into their homes and the world, these formal rules have the appearance of giving an official status to the simple mechanics of well-baby care that were once determined by common sense.

Those doctors, nurses, and grandparents who create rules for the care of newborns often do so using the pretense of helping mothers to learn the proper management of their infants and to make them feel more secure while they are learning their new job. But the rules often have the opposite effect. The greater the number of rules, the more reliant the mother has to become on her teacher (thereby making the teacher more important), and the more insecure the mother may become. Moreover, the reason that so many baby books offer parents conflicting advice concerning tthe baby's health or well being.

In most cases, it makes little difference whether the baby is fed on demand or on a strict schedule (mothers whose personalities are very relaxed prefer demand feedings while those whose personalities are more structured generally prefer a formal schedule). A waiting time before taking the baby outside is not usually necessary (if it is all right to take the baby from the hospital to the house in a January snowstorm, there is no reason that the baby cannot go outside again if it is properly dressed and protected). Also, it makes little difference whether the baby is started on rice cereal or bananas as the first food. If a few days between new foods are allowed, it will be easy to discover a food that does not agree with the baby.

It is clear that the best advice for new parents is to read different books, talk to friends and relatives, and ask for information that may be useful to them when they are taking care of their new baby. Advice should be viewed by parents as a *guide* that may or may not be useful depending on their life-styles and personalities. New mothers and fathers should get used to making decisions and taking responsibility for the care of their child from the beginning rather than allow someone else to make the decisions for them. Common sense should take priority over the rules someone else has made, which may have applied to their own home setting but may not necessarily apply to your situation at home.

143

UNDERSTANDING YOUR FEELINGS

One of the most exciting experiences of your lifetime is bringing your new baby home from the hospital. It is a time when fears about the baby developing normally have usually disappeared and there is the excitement of thinking about your baby as your offspring. For the first time, the husband and wife are *truly* related to each other, and their family has been created.

Many mothers, however, do not expect the feelings of nervousness, anxiety, and occasional depression that are often felt soon after the baby is born. Although these feelings are common, most mothers do not discuss them with friends because they feel guilty about having negative thoughts at a time when they are expected to be very happy. Why do these feelings occur?

First, a mother's body undergoes the same physiological changes after a baby is born that occur just before her menstrual period. The high hormone levels necessary to maintain the pregnancy drop off suddenly after the baby is born, just as they do immediately before menstruation begins. Those mothers who normally feel tense, depressed, or tearful before the onset of their period may have similar feelings shortly after the birth of their baby.

Second, having a baby is the start of a new job. Often parents feel insecure about doing everything properly. They are receiving advice from friends and relatives, and although they want to be independent, they are not sure which advice to accept and which to reject.

Third, the mother may be overtired. Giving birth to a baby requires a lot of energy, and the added pressures of entertaining visitors, getting up for middle-of-the-night feedings, and having a regular schedule disrupted by the baby's cranky periods, nap times, and feedings can easily create a situation where she finds herself disorganized and weary.

In addition, some mothers feel they have been displaced from the center of attention. Before the baby is born, they receive calls regularly asking if they are feeling well. After the baby is born, the callers (and often the fathers) ask only how the baby is, just at the time when the mothers would like someone to be thinking about them most.

It is not surprising, therefore, that some mothers find themselves alone and crying while everyone is telling them how proud and happy they should be feeling. Generally, the feelings of happiness that surround the birth of the baby will usually be much stronger than those depressed feelings described above. The negative feelings are discussed here because a mother may not understand why her tearful episodes occur and she may then feel guilty about them. This may cause even more nervousness if she doesn't realize that these thoughts are normal and natural. More importantly, these feelings should not be allowed to detract from the fun and pleasure of watching the baby grow and develop.

HOW TO PREPARE OLDER CHILDREN FOR THE NEW BABY

To make older children feel at ease about a new baby being brought into the house, parents will often play down the role the new brother or sister will have in the family. They may also try to make the older child feel important at the expense of their new sibling. These tactics may be reflected by such statements as "Boy, isn't that baby a nuisance! I wish he wouldn't cry so much." Or, "The baby is really awful. He needs to be held all the time." When someone comes into the room and remarks that the baby is cute, these parents will usually glance toward the older child, indicating to the visitor that he should be quiet. If you have more than one previous child, read the section on the Middle Child Syndrome.

The problem with this approach to avoiding jealousy is that it creates hatred in its place. Why should the older child have a desire to protect, like, or want to be friends with his new sibling if everyone acts as though the new baby isn't important and is not worth having around? While it is reasonable to let the older child know that he can do certain things that the baby cannot because he is older, it should never be indicated to him that he is better because he is older. If he is taught that he is better rather than different, the distinction will become especially obvious when the children are older and the first child becomes physically and verbally abusive to the second.

It is much more reasonable to insist that the older child treat the new baby with respect as a new family member, and allow him to act out or discuss honestly any feelings of jealousy. The parents can help by making remarks that let the child know that they understand his feelings and that those feelings are all right as long as he does not take them out on the new baby. "I know that you feel upset because everyone has been giving a lot of attention to the new baby. That is happening because everyone is welcoming him into our family. This is really like his first birthday. We did the same thing for you when you came into our family." "I know that you are upset because I can't come now. I feel badly too, but the baby can't eat without my help." (Note the difference from "Go away! I'm feeding the baby.")

In general, if you want the baby to be treated with respect by your older child you must do the same.

USING THE TELEPHONE

COMMON COMPLAINTS

MINOR INFECTIONS

INFECTIOUS DISEASES

EMERGENCY PROBLEMS

NEW INFANT CARE

PEDIATRIC PROBLEMS

145

USING THE
TELEPHONE

COMMON
COMPLAINTS

MINOR
INFECTIONS

INFECTIOUS
DISEASES

EMERGENCY
PROBLEMS

NEW INFANT
CARE

PEDIATRIC
PROBLEMS

BREAST- VS. BOTTLE-FEEDING

If you do not have a strong preference for breast- or bottle-feeding, begin by breast-feeding and change to formula if you find it unpleasant or not practical. It is difficult to make the change in reverse.

Breast-feeding has many biochemical and physiological advantages over bottle-feeding. At least as important, however, is that the feeding should be enjoyable to the mother as well as to the baby. When nursing goes well and is found to be pleasurable by the mother, it is without question the preferred method of providing nutrition for the baby.

If a mother has *strong* reservations about breast-feeding, she should not feel guilty about choosing a prepared formula. The potential medical disadvantages of bottle-feeding (most of which are minor) are not nearly as great a disadvantage to the baby as having its mother dread each feeding if she dislikes putting the baby to breast. A mother should choose the type of feeding *she* believes is best for her and her baby. The choice should not be made by someone else for her.

BREAST-FEEDING

During the first few days, many mothers have little milk, and many infants feed poorly. However, within a short period of time you and your baby will adjust to a reasonable feeding schedule.

Guide the baby's mouth to your breast by holding his head from behind. Avoid pushing his cheek with your hand, since by reflex he will turn toward the pressure rather than toward your breast. Because the milk is squeezed from the breast, place as much of the areola (colored part surrounding the nipple) in the baby's mouth as possible. If only the tip of the nipple is offered, soreness and poor feeding will follow.

If the baby has difficulty taking the breast because it is engorged (swollen), express a small amount of milk by pressing the areola between two fingers before the baby begins feeding. Similarly, if engorgement occurs because the baby has missed a feeding, the same procedure may be used. The baby's suction should be broken before removing him from the breast by placing a finger in the corner of his mouth.

The following schedule may be used as a guide for the initial breast-feedings. Some infants feed more quickly than others, however, so don't be afraid to alter it for your baby.

146

Day 1:	First breast		5 min.,	Second breast		5 min.
Day 2:	"	"	5 min.,	"	"	10 min.
Day 3:	"	"	10 min.,	"	"	10 min.
Day 4:	"	"	10 min.,	"	"	15 min.
Day 5:	"	"	10 min.,	"	"	20 min.

USING THE TELEPHONE

COMMON COMPLAINTS

MINOR INFECTIONS

INFECTIOUS DISEASES

EMERGENCY PROBLEMS

NEW INFANT CARE

PEDIATRIC PROBLEMS

Alternate the starting breast at each feeding. A safety pin may be placed on the bra strap at the starting side as a reminder.

Sore nipples are best treated with a bland ointment such as A & D. Air drying at frequent intervals is most important. This may be accomplished by holding loose-fitting clothing away from your body.

During the first week breast-feed your infant as frequently as is practical to increase your milk supply. When your infant seems constantly hungry, either sugar water or formula may be offered to your baby immediately after your breast-feeding has been completed. Do not offer formula between feedings as this will decrease your milk supply. When the baby no longer seems interested in this after-feeding bottle, or is taking only a small amount, its use may be discontinued. This will supplement your baby's calories and fluids until your milk has come in completely. If desired, one *supplemental* bottle may be offered instead of one breast-feeding each day. Supplemental bottles allow the father to participate in feedings, allow you to leave the baby with a sitter, and permit occasional change-off for middle-of-the-night feedings.

While breast-feeding, try to eat a balanced diet and to drink additional fluids to replace those being given to the baby. All foods are acceptable if eaten in moderation. However, if your eating a food repeatedly causes your baby to be irritable, avoit it in the future. Large amounts of chocolate and caffeine (cola, tea, and coffee) are common offenders. Do not take medications, including laxatives, unless your doctor is contacted first.

Although breast milk usually contains adequate amounts of vitamins, the quantity may vary from feeding to feeding and your doctor may recommend that vitamin drops be given to the baby. Schedules for feedings will be discussed later in this chapter.

Call the doctor on a nonurgent basis if:

1. Your nipples become cracked or so painful that it is difficult to feed the baby.
2. You develop a breast infection or other illness, especially if you have fever.
3. You are considering taking medicines of any kind.
4. Your baby always appears hungry, is completely unscheduled, appears to be losing weight, or wets his diaper infrequently.

USING THE TELEPHONE

COMMON COMPLAINTS

MINOR INFECTIONS

INFECTIOUS DISEASES

EMERGENCY PROBLEMS

NEW INFANT CARE

PEDIATRIC PROBLEMS

FORMULA-FEEDING

Most pediatricians believe that formula containing iron should be given to your baby during the first year of life. Although the iron contained in formula is frequently blamed for constipation, colic, and other complaints, changing to formula that does not contain iron usually makes little difference.

If *ready-to-use formulas* are chosen, sterilization of the bottles and nipples is not necessary. The top of the can containing the formula should be washed prior to opening and should be covered before storage in the refrigerator. Formula may be poured into bottles that have been washed thoroughly before use, but they need not be sterile if the formula is fed to the baby within two to three hours after filling. Unused formula should be discarded within forty-eight hours to prevent spoilage.

If a *concentrated formula* is chosen, it provides a convenient way of giving fluoride to your baby to prevent later tooth decay when your local water supply is fluoridated. *Terminal sterilization* is the procedure of choice for preparing concentrated formula. After filling the bottles halfway with formula, you should add tap water until the bottle is completely full. The nipples should then be inverted into the bottle and all of the bottles for the day should be placed in a sterilizer rack. This entire package—bottles, nipples, formula, and water—should be boiled for twenty minutes. The bottles can then be refrigerated and warmed individually by running hot tap water over them just before giving them to the baby. Although it has been conventional for the day's formula to be made in early morning hours, there is no reason why the full day's supply of bottles cannot be prepared at midday or in the evening hours.

Formulas are also available in throwaway, prepackaged *individual bottles.* Generally this is an expensive way to feed the baby, but it is a major advantage when going on trips or leaving the baby with a babysitter. This prepackaged formula can be kept at room temperature and does not have to be warmed. Most infants prefer formula that has been brought to a medium *temperature,* but chilled formula will not harm the baby.

Prepared formulas contain the infant's daily required vitamins, so vitamin supplements are not necessary. Supplemental vitamins should be offered, however, when formula feeding is discontinued.

FEEDING SCHEDULES

As discussed earlier, mothers who live their lives in a very orderly fashion will find that a *formal schedule* of every three or four hours will fit best into their daily routines. Those mothers whose days are lived in a less structured way may find that feeding their babies on *demand* whenever they are hungry will make both baby and mother feel most comfortable. Making a compromise between a formal schedule and a demand schedule has proved to be best for most mothers, however:

During the day, avoid feeding babies more frequently than at three-hour intervals to avoid the possibility of their taking one ounce an hour instead of three ounces every three hours. Allowing the baby to sleep longer than four hours during the day without feeding may also be unwise, since the baby might fall into a schedule of sleeping all day and then being up all night. During the nighttime, infants should be fed only if they awaken spontaneously. When babies require food during nighttime hours, they will not let you forget them.

SOLID FOODS

The age at which small babies should be started on solid foods is a matter of controversy but there is general agreement that during the early months breast milk or formula is the best, most balanced source of nutrition. Solid foods are often begun early because of pressure from relatives, boredom from giving the baby nothing but milk to drink, and as an attempt to get the baby to sleep through the night. Most infants will not sleep through the night until ten to twelve weeks of age regardless of when solid foods are started. Although most infants will reflexively suck on a nipple shortly after birth, most will also push food out of their mouth by reflex until they are about this age. Many pediatricians believe that this reflex has the purpose of telling the parent that the baby is not ready to begin solids yet. Early introduction of solid foods also has the disadvantage of offering the baby a diet that is not properly balanced and may increase difficulties with bowel movements, digestion, and possible allergic reactions.

A compromise to the conflicting recommendations concerning the feeding of solid foods is to start with bland, strained foods when the baby weighs approximately 15 pounds. At this stage most infants are taking approximately eight ounces of milk at a feeding, and solids will provide an alternate to giving more than eight ounces at any given time. Two tablespoons of solid food replace one ounce of breast milk or formula. It is reasonable to start the baby with a bland food such as rice cereal, applesauce, or banana once or twice a day. Because most infants prefer

USING THE TELEPHONE

COMMON COMPLAINTS

MINOR INFECTIONS

INFECTIOUS DISEASES

EMERGENCY PROBLEMS

NEW INFANT CARE

PEDIATRIC PROBLEMS

149

USING THE
TELEPHONE

COMMON
COMPLAINTS

MINOR
INFECTIONS

INFECTIOUS
DISEASES

EMERGENCY
PROBLEMS

NEW INFANT
CARE

PEDIATRIC
PROBLEMS

to suck rather than eat, three or four ounces of milk is usually given first. This followed by solid food, which in turn is followed by more milk. At least two to three days should be allowed between the introduction of one new food and the next so that intolerance or allergies will be more noticeable.

It has been suggested that mixing sweet fruits with bland cereals does not allow your infant to develop a taste for unsweetened foods. Although these two foods may be given at the same feeding, they should not be mixed together on the spoon or added to the baby's milk. In recent years, mothers have become interested in preparing pureed foods for their babies in preference to giving brand-name strained foods. This practice is perfectly acceptable as long as the homemade foods given to the infant do not have salt or sugar added to "improve" their flavor.

WEANING YOUR INFANT FROM THE BREAST

Although breast milk is preferred to other milk forms during the first year of life, mothers frequently find that it is not practical to breast-feed for that length of time. The most important medical advantages to breast-feeding take place during the first 3 months of life and many mothers choose to wean their infants at that time. Six months is another common time for weaning because babies are taking solid foods and because first teeth erupt at this age.

The American Academy of Pediatrics has recommended that infants be weaned to an infant formula rather than to cow's milk until the baby is *one year old*. This recommendation was made because the protein in prepared infant formulas is more easily digested than the protein contained in cow's milk; the formula protein is less likely to irritate the baby's bowel resulting in small amounts of food loss; minerals such as calcium and phosphorus have been adjusted in the formula to be more similar to the amounts found in breast milk; and the salt content of formula is lower than that found in cow's milk, possibly decreasing the chances of the baby developing high blood pressure at a later age. In addition, when the formula is fortified with iron, which is found in very small quantities in cow's milk, there is less likelihood of the baby developing iron deficiency anemia during this period of very rapid growth.

Although most mothers wean their infants by skipping one breast-feeding every 3 or 4 days and substituting a bottle for the missed feeding, this method causes much discomfort. The breast engorgement which follows the missed feedings can only be partially relieved by wearing a tight bra or binder, applying either heat or cold (whichever feels best), and taking pain relieving medicines.

A more practical approach to weaning is one of shortening the period of breast-feeding and then following the breast-feeding with a bottle of formula. If the usual breast-feeding period is 30 minutes, shorten it to 25 minutes for 2 or 3 days, then 20 minutes, and so on. In this way the baby will gradually take more and more of his feeding from the bottle while allowing your breast milk supply to decrease gradually.

CARE OF THE UMBILICUS (BELLY BUTTON)

The belly button scab should be treated in much the same way as a scab at any other location on the body. That is, it should be exposed to the air as much as possible and an attempt should be made to keep the area clean. The upper portion of the diaper should be left below the belly button so that the belly button may dry out sooner. When the scab falls off, some bleeding or oozing may be noted and additional drying of the area can be accomplished by applying alcohol with a cotton swab. If the belly button area has constant oozing, a foul smell, a pussy discharge, or is surrounded by an area of redness, these signs may indicate an infection and your physician should be called for advice.

BATHING

When the belly button scab has healed, the infant may be placed in a tub or sink containing lukewarm water for a proper bath. Before that time, sponge bathing is recommended daily or every second day. A bland soap such as castile should be used, but care should be taken to completely rinse it from the skin to prevent excessive drying, especially during winter months.

CARE OF THE SKIN

An infant's skin should be treated in much the same manner an adult would treat her own. If the skin is dry, a baby lotion should be applied as a moistening agent. If the baby develops a heat rash, talcum powder or cornstarch may be applied to absorb perspiration. If the baby's skin appears normal, no special care is necessary.

151

USING THE TELEPHONE

COMMON COMPLAINTS

MINOR INFECTIONS

INFECTIOUS DISEASES

EMERGENCY PROBLEMS

NEW INFANT CARE

PEDIATRIC PROBLEMS

USING THE TELEPHONE

COMMON COMPLAINTS

MINOR INFECTIONS

INFECTIOUS DISEASES

EMERGENCY PROBLEMS

NEW INFANT CARE

PEDIATRIC PROBLEMS

The skin covered by the diaper may be protected from urine and stools by applying a thin coat of petroleum jelly with each diaper change. Mild rashes in the diaper area should be treated by allowing the skin to air dry. You may with to pin the diaper to the front and the back of the baby's shirt while leaving the sides open so that most of the urine and stool will be retained but air will still be allowed to enter.

Many infants develop rashes on their cheeks during the first few weeks of life. These rashes may look like acne and can be caused by hormones that have crossed to the baby, by sheets from which detergent has not been thoroughly removed during rinsing, or by allowing the baby's cheeks to rub against wool sweaters or coats worn by the parents. These rashes may appear and disappear throughout the day, usually looking worse after the infant awakens from a nap. Because they often disappear without treatment, no special skin care is necessary. However, if the rash looks particularly severe, applying a mild hydrocortisone cream (which may be purchased without prescription) will often provide rapid improvement.

Additional information may be found in the section on Diaper rash (p. 71).

BOWEL MOVEMENTS

The frequency and consistency of a baby's stools often vary on a day-to-day basis. Some babies have a movement after each feeding while others may pass a stool once a day or once every two days. Breast-fed babies tend to have more frequent and looser stools than those made by bottle-fed babies, and it is not uncommon for them to leak from the diaper at the time of the feeding.

When stools are thought to consist almost entirely of water with very little solid material, and these watery stools occur three or four times in a row, they should be reported to your physician because they may represent diarrhea. If stools are so hard that they form little pebbles and this becomes your infant's usual pattern, it should also be reported to your doctor, since this represents constipation. Those stools that are pasty, seedy, or have the consistency of heavy cream or pea soup are all perfectly normal.

Although green stools tend to cause major concern to most parents, they mean only that it has passed through the infant's bowel so quickly that the bile contained within the stool has not changed color from green to brown or yellow. Straining while having a bowel movement also causes concern to many parents, but if the stool appears normal, straining does not indicate a problem for the baby.

Additional information may be found in the section on Diarrhea (p. 57) and Constipation (p. 61).

TAKING THE BABY OUT

If your baby is dressed properly, he may be taken out of the house at any time. Since there was no problem when bringing the baby from the hospital to your home, there is no reason to expect that a problem will arise from taking the baby out a few days later. However, if the trip is not necessary, it is suggested that planned walks be started when the baby is one or two weeks old depending on your physical condition and the weather.

VISITORS DURING THE BABY'S INFANCY

Part of the enjoyment of having a new baby is sharing it with close friends and relatives. However, people with colds and illnesses should avoid contact if at all possible. Do not allow a large number of people to handle the baby. It makes good sense to limit those who do have close contact to two or three friends and relatives.

SMOKING NEAR THE BABY

While it is common knowledge that mothers who smoke during pregnancy may have smaller infants, it is not commonly known that infants whose parents smoke may have a two to three times higher incidence of bronchitis and pneumonia during the first year because of irritation from the cigarette smoke. For that reason, parents and visitors should smoke cigarettes in areas that will not be occupied by the infant during the following two to three hours. No one should be permitted to smoke in the baby's room.

TRAVELING WITH THE BABY

All infants should be strapped into an approved car restraint at all times. Car beds do not provide the infant with any protection during an automobile accident. Traveling with the infant on one's lap can be just as dangerous. If it is absolutely necessary to travel while holding the baby, sit in the rear seat.

153

USING THE TELEPHONE

COMMON COMPLAINTS

MINOR INFECTIONS

INFECTIOUS DISEASES

EMERGENCY PROBLEMS

NEW INFANT CARE

PEDIATRIC PROBLEMS

USING THE TELEPHONE

COMMON COMPLAINTS

MINOR INFECTIONS

INFECTIOUS DISEASES

EMERGENCY PROBLEMS

NEW INFANT CARE

PEDIATRIC PROBLEMS

WATCHING YOUR BABY GROW

One of the most exciting rewards of parenthood is watching your baby grow and develop. When you bring your infant to her physician for "well-baby" visits, the doctor will discuss the baby's nutrition and development with you. However, a baby who sits, walks, and talks earlier than average will not necessarily be smarter than average, nor will a baby who performs these tasks more slowly necessarily be less smart when she grows up. Large babies are not necessarily large adults and small babies born to tall parents are not the least bit uncommon.

Following your baby's growth and development is very useful as a *rough guide* that she is progressing well, but it should not be used as a way for predicting how things will go in the future. Do not make the mistake of wishing away your baby's "babyhood." Too many parents "can't wait" until the baby rolls, sits, or walks, and miss the enjoyment of what she is doing *now*. The result is that they suddenly realize they have missed a lot of fun.

Parents who have more than one child usually learn this important lesson and conclude that it is perfectly all right if the baby remains babyish just a little longer.

IMMUNIZATIONS

The following immunization schedule has been recommended by the American Academy of Pediatrics. Some pediatricians use a schedule which is somewhat different. You should discuss it with your doctor at the "well baby" visit.

2 months	DPT (diphtheria, pertussis, tetanus)
	TOPV (trivalent oral polio vaccine)
4 months	DPT, TOPV
6 months	DPT
12 months	Tuberculin test
15 months	Measles, rubella, mumps
18 months	DPT, TOPV
4–6 years	DPT, TOPV
14–16 years	DT (diphtheria and tetanus)—repeat every 10 years

Reactions to immunizations

DPT (diphtheria, pertussis, tetanus)
    Reactions:
    Fever lasting a few hours to twenty-four hours. Redness and swelling at the site of injection. Irritability or drowsiness.
    Treatment:
    Aspirin or acetaminophen for fever and irritability; cool compresses on the site of injection.

TOPV (trivalent oral polio vaccine)
    Reactions:
    Occasional loose or diarrheal stools
    Treatment:
    None
DT (diphtheria and tetanus)
    Reactions:
    Local tenderness at the site of injection.
    Treatment:
    Cool compresses applied locally.

USING THE TELEPHONE

COMMON COMPLAINTS

MINOR INFECTIONS

INFECTIOUS DISEASES

EMERGENCY PROBLEMS

NEW INFANT CARE

PEDIATRIC PROBLEMS

Measles
Reactions:
Upper respiratory tract infection.
Cough, fever, and/or rash resembling measles that appears 5 to 10 days after the immunization has been received.
Treatment:
Aspirin for fever. The rash usually does not cause other symptoms and is not contagious. It does not require treatment.

Mumps
Reactions:
Upper respiratory tract infection. Occasional low-grade fever 7 to 10 days after injection.
Treatment:
Aspirin for fever.

Rubella (German measles)
Reactions:
A generalized measles-like rash. Joint pain in older individuals may be noted 5 to 10 days after the injection.
Treatment:
Aspirin to relieve symptoms.

MMR (measles, mumps, and rubella)
Reactions:
Upper respiratory tract infection with fever and/or cough. Generalized measles-like rash appearing 5 to 10 days after the injection.
Treatment:
Aspirin for fever.
No isolation is necessary for individuals with rash as it is not considered contagious.

COMMON CONCERNS REGARDING NEWBORNS

Irregular Breathing

Do not be concerned if your baby has uneven or erratic breathing patterns during the first few months of life as long as the infant otherwise appears well and has good color. Noisy breathing is also usual for most babies.

Bowing of the Legs

A curve of the lower legs may be seen during the first few months because of the way the baby's legs were held before birth. The curvature will be seen at the place where one leg crossed over the other during the time the baby was in the fetal position.

Red Marks Above the Eyes and the Back of the Neck

This reddish discoloration of the skin is normal and is commonly referred to as "stork bites." These will usually disappear without treatment before the baby's first birthday.

Puffy Eyes

Many hospitals place silver nitrate drops in the baby's eyes at birth to prevent certain types of eye infections. These drops have an irritating effect and may cause eye swelling or discharge that disappears after a few days. If the swelling or discharge lasts longer, call your doctor.

Crossed Eyes

Because newborn infants do not see well at a distance and cannot fix on objects, their eyes may occasionally cross. Also, babies have

USING THE TELEPHONE

COMMON COMPLAINTS

MINOR INFECTIONS

INFECTIOUS DISEASES

EMERGENCY PROBLEMS

NEW INFANT CARE

PEDIATRIC PROBLEMS

USING THE
TELEPHONE

COMMON
COMPLAINTS

MINOR
INFECTIONS

INFECTIOUS
DISEASES

EMERGENCY
PROBLEMS

NEW INFANT
CARE

PEDIATRIC
PROBLEMS

a wide bridge to their nose which may make their eyes appear crossed when in fact they are not. Discuss the appearance of crossed eyes with your doctor at the time of the first well-baby examination.

Yellow Jaundice

Until the baby's liver begins to make the right enzymes and function properly, many infants develop a yellow color to their skin as a pigment called bilirubin is deposited within it. Slight yellow color to the skin, especially around the nose, is normal. If your baby looks obviously yellow or orange, call your doctor immediately for advice.

Cradle Cap

A yellow, oily crusting of the scalp is frequently seen during the first few months. Since this represents a baby's version of dandruff, nonprescription dandruff shampoos will usually be effective for treatment.

Coated Tongue

See the section "Thrush."

Chapter VIII
COMMON PEDIATRIC AND PSYCHOLOGICAL PROBLEMS

USING THE TELEPHONE

COMMON COMPLAINTS

MINOR INFECTIONS

INFECTIOUS DISEASES

EMERGENCY PROBLEMS

NEW INFANT CARE

PEDIATRIC PROBLEMS

159

USING THE TELEPHONE

COMMON COMPLAINTS

MINOR INFECTIONS

INFECTIOUS DISEASES

EMERGENCY PROBLEMS

NEW INFANT CARE

PEDIATRIC PROBLEMS

USING THE TELEPHONE

COMMON COMPLAINTS

MINOR INFECTIONS

INFECTIOUS DISEASES

EMERGENCY PROBLEMS

NEW INFANT CARE

COMMON COMPLAINTS LISTED BY AGE GROUP

Not all children develop at the same rate. Some will socialize and talk before others, while the slow socializers may learn their motor skills (sitting, walking, running) very quickly. The rate of development of these skills may have some influence on your baby's early "personality," but most pediatricians agree that babies also appear to have intrinsic differences in personality that are obvious even during the first few weeks and months.

The differences in parents' personalities and in babies' personalities and development make each baby-parent grouping different. In much the same way that parents' attitudes toward the baby will have an effect on the baby, the baby's personality may have a major effect on the parent. It is much easier for a mother to be affectionate, loving, and relaxed toward a cuddly, smiling, relaxed baby than toward a baby who is frequently cranky, irritable, and difficult to feed. These intrinsic differences *must* be considered when you compare your baby to someone else's. Your parenting experience may be completely different from theirs even though the babies are the same age.

Many parental concerns about children's behavior are really concerns over their *normal* development, however. The most common "problems" are outlined below.

One month:

Stomach pain: See Chapter II, "Stomach Pain in Infants" (p. 50).

Three months

Teething: Your baby's teeth usually won't appear until six months of age, when the two middle bottom teeth first erupt. However, at about two and a half or three months of age most infants will start to show signs of early teething. Babies will frequently bite on their fists and drool more often than in the past. Many infants will also have a wet cough, which is more noticeable in the morning as they attempt to clear the saliva which has

USING THE TELEPHONE

COMMON COMPLAINTS

MINOR INFECTIONS

INFECTIOUS DISEASES

EMERGENCY PROBLEMS

NEW INFANT CARE

PEDIATRIC PROBLEMS

settled in the back of their throats. This morning cough may be mistaken for a cold, but when no runny nose is seen, it is most likely the result of this early teething process.

Six months

Crying episodes: Crying, waking up during the night, and fretfulness while sleeping frequently begin at about six months as babies actually cut their first two teeth. Many topical anesthetics to numb the gums are available in the local pharmacy. Unfortunately, most of them offer relief that doesn't last more than five or ten minutes.

Giving your baby aspirin or acetaminophen may be useful because these pain-relievers are effective for three to four hours. If you rub your baby's gums with just your dry finger he will often find relief and will be able to return to sleep. Do not let your baby sleep with a bottle in his mouth since either milk, formula, or juice will bathe his new teeth for long periods during sleep and severe tooth decay may occur.

Seven months:

Extra attention is needed when babies are first able to creep and pull themselves to standing. They begin to think of their playpens or cribs as restricting their activity. Many will therefore protest when you leave them alone even for short periods. Parents frequently will treat a baby's crying when left alone as a sign of spoiled behavior when in fact it represents the baby's frustration at not being able to come along. Spend as much time with your child as is practical but do not feel guilty for allowing your child to cry on occasion.

Twelve to fifteen months

Poor eating: See the section on poor eating later in this chapter.

Fifteen months to two and a half years

Frequent temper tantrums and poor eating habits: Temper tantrums at this age may be the result of your child being able to understand much more of what is going on around him than he is able to express. This

162

inability to tell what he knows may finally result in his throwing himself down on the ground and screaming or crying. When these temper tantrums do occur, you should try to give your youngster as little attention as possible so that he will have less incentive to repeat them the next time. After the tantrum is ended, you may wish to pick up your child and be affectionate as a way of rewarding him for having stopped this behavior, and as a reminder that you still love him.

Many children in this age group have a *negative attitude* toward doing things you want them to do. They may suddenly resent getting dressed or undressed, taking a bath or coming out of the tub, and other such normal daytime activities. The common mistake made by many parents is to believe that a long discussion pointing out the reasons for doing something will make their child more cooperative. However, most children at this age are simply not reasonable during these discussions. A forceful but friendly parent is usually more effective. It is sometimes helpful with first children to make believe that you have another child who requires your attention while you are dressing your eighteen-month-old, to determine how much time should really be spent with him. Most children at this age are very forgiving and in most cases, five or ten minutes after you've dressed or bathed your child against his will, he will no longer seem upset by the incident.

While within this age group children tend to eat less at mealtime than previously, one good meal per day with many small nutritious snacks is a normal eating pattern. (See the section on Eating Problems.)

Ages two-and-one-half to three-and-one-half

Variable behavior: Periods of cooperative behavior alternating with cranky, irritable, demanding, and compulsive behavior are usual at this age. Bedtime and eating rituals, with occasional outbursts of temper when things do not go the child's way, are also common. Many of these children are able to do a large number of the things required of them in daily routine, including making conversation, feeding and dressing themselves, and getting around the house without difficulty. However because they are not really proficient at performing these skills, they may feel insecure about doing many of them. Just as an adult tries to arrange a desk carefully when starting a new job so that an emergency will be easier to handle, small children will carefully arrange stuffed animals before going to bed, insist that a sandwich be cut in only one direction, have a temper tantrum if the peas get mixed with the potatoes, or become very upset when daily routines are changed. You can help your child by

USING THE TELEPHONE

COMMON COMPLAINTS

MINOR INFECTIONS

INFECTIOUS DISEASES

EMERGENCY PROBLEMS

NEW INFANT CARE

PEDIATRIC PROBLEMS

163

USING THE TELEPHONE

COMMON COMPLAINTS

MINOR INFECTIONS

INFECTIOUS DISEASES

EMERGENCY PROBLEMS

NEW INFANT CARE

PEDIATRIC PROBLEMS

making his day as predictable as is practical and by understanding the reasons for his frustration. In addition, the child's mood swings may coincide with similar mood swings of the parents. When you feel tense, irritable, and depressed, you may have less patience for your child's problems and become short-tempered with him, thus making him tense, irritable, and depressed. Likewise, if your child is upset and very demanding of your time, you might find yourself feeling very nervous in your response to his actions. When you begin to feel edgy, allow yourself scheduled time off just as you would from any other job. Knowing that you have free time on a particular morning or afternoon will make your week much more tolerable when you are feeling tired or depressed.

This period is one of the *most* frustrating for parents to deal with. A parent is willing to accept temperamental, babyish behavior before their children are speaking well, but once they become verbal and can express themselves, the children appear more "mature." At this point, the impulsive mood swings and frustrations that are seen in many three-year-olds become *very* difficult to deal with. In addition to the suggestions contained in the section "What to Do When Your Child Has Behavior Problems" (pp. 166–168), you simply have to "hang in there" until your child gets older.

Ages three-and-one-half to four-and-one-half

Demanding, asks many questions, insists on doing things by himself: Children of this age are especially interested in learning about the things around them and are very insistent that you provide them with as much information as they are capable of learning. They will not be satisfied with partial answers to questions or evasions. When a four-year-old shouts to his mother, "Mommy, where are you?" and his mother responds, "I'll be there in a minute," the child may answer "Yes, but where are you?"

These children are also intent on forcing you to allow them to practice skills they are just learning. For this reason, a four-year-old will often not be at all concerned that you are late for an appointment while he is busy buckling his belt by himself. The greatest frustration to parents comes when the children put you in the impossible situation of first being angry at you when you try to help them perform a task, and then becoming angry at you when they cannot do it alone. Many parents find this Catch-22 maddening, but it becomes more tolerable when you realize the child is as frustrated as you are.

164

Ages six to seven

Talking back and being angry at parents: Many first-graders feel angry at having to conform to strict rules imposed on them by their teachers. This is the first school year when the children have to sit at their desks, do their work by their teacher's rules, and comply with someone else's wishes in a regimented situation for almost an entire day. It is not uncommon for them to be angry at their parents for putting them in this situation. When expressing anger to their parents at home, however, children usually do not mention school. They will frequently complain about their lunch, the clothes they are wearing, or an activity that was planned for later in the day. Understanding that anger expressed toward parents may really be a reflection of difficulties that the child is having at school or with friends will make this time much easier for the parents.

Ages seven to nine

Pressure from friends to conform: It is normal for children to want to conform to their group of friends, but this desire may cause unexplained mood swings if your child is having difficulty within his social group. Problems relating to learning school material may also present psychological problems in this age group, since some children may use attention-getting behavior as a means of drawing attention away from their difficulty with reading or mathematics. If your seven- to nine-year-old seems especially unhappy at home, contacting his teacher and checking on his academic progress and his relations with other children may provide some clues to the reasons for that unhappiness.

Ages ten to twelve

Mood changes and "doesn't feel like doing anything": Many pre-teenagers find themselves in a situation similar to that of the middle child. They are reprimanded for doing things that seem too childish but then are told they are not old enough when they try to act like teenagers. Finding themselves in this middle ground, these children tend to withdraw from activities they previously liked and may have difficulty coordinating their interests. For that reason, parents should try to promote activities that stress their children's strengths rather than encouraging them to be "well-rounded" during this stage of development. A cynical parent recently suggested to me that the reason children seem especially moody during their early teen years is that they are preparing for adulthood.

165

USING THE TELEPHONE

COMMON COMPLAINTS

MINOR INFECTIONS

INFECTIOUS DISEASES

EMERGENCY PROBLEMS

NEW INFANT CARE

PEDIATRIC PROBLEMS

USING THE
TELEPHONE

COMMON
COMPLAINTS

MINOR
INFECTIONS

INFECTIOUS
DISEASES

EMERGENCY
PROBLEMS

NEW INFANT
CARE

PEDIATRIC
PROBLEMS

WHAT TO DO
WHEN YOUR CHILD HAS
BEHAVIOR PROBLEMS:

What the doctor needs to know:

1. Duration: Has the problem been going on for a long time or is it relatively recent?
2. Frequency: Is your child having problems in just one area of social contact (home, school, and friends) or does it affect all those areas?
3. Family problems: Have there been any recent problems at home (money-related, fighting, a drinking problem, etc.)?
4. Cause: Although you may not know the exact cause of the problem, if you had to pick one thing you think is responsible, what would you choose?

Discussion:

Many of the problems parents believe should be discussed with their physician are related to normal childhood development. Usually these are difficulties with management of day-to-day life rather than true problems your child is facing. The most common ones have just been discussed by age group in the preceding section.

When you believe that a problem is chronic (going on for a long time and likely to continue) or if it includes all areas of your child's activities (family, work, and friends), you should definitely contact your physician or a trained professional to discuss your child's problems at length. Do not assume that a problem that has continued for three or four years or one that has made your child unhappy with respect to all areas of his functioning, and allows him no place to take refuge, will go away by itself. You must actively investigate its cause.

In order to convert your child's difficulties into a problem for which you will be able to find workable solutions, the following advice should prove useful:

1. *Delineate the problem:* Choose three or four of the most troublesome kinds of behavior and think about ways of solving them while ignoring less important problems. Separating out these especially difficult areas may help to give you the feeling that there are *specific* things you can do instead of having a general impression that "things are not going well."

2. *Establish the causative factors:* Review all the major family difficulties of the past year that may have had a major influence on your child. These would include: a parent who has lost a job, a child who has changed schools, friends who have moved away, or a death in the family. These episodes may not be directly responsible for your child's problem, but they are possibly contributing to it.

3. *Question your child:* Your child himself may be the best source of information concerning what's bothering him—ask him. Parents frequently forget to ask their child about his problems in a straightforward way. You should not be threatening or use a manner which accuses him as if the problem were his fault. The questions should be asked in a way that gives him the feeling that you understand his problems and truly wish to help him. For example, you might say "I've been feeling badly for you. I can see that things haven't being going well. Is there anything you'd like to talk to me about?"

4. *Take time off:* Being a full-time parent is mentally and physically strenuous. As with other jobs, having time off to think about yourself is important to keeping yourself productive and good-spirited. When the relationship between a parent and a young child is not going well, the parent may respond by feeling guilty and leave the child with another person less often. This is a mistake, since the problem will only become worse unless a regularly scheduled "mini-vacation" time is chosen.

5. *Develop a punishment:* It is absolutely essential that an effective punishment be chosen as a means of maintaining discipline. The punishment you select will depend on the age of your youngster and on both his personality and yours. Hitting should be reserved for infrequent special occasions, and separating your child from the others around him for even a short period may prove to be more effective. If he is going to be placed in another room, he should be told that he has been separated because of something that he did and not because you wish it that way. Statements such as "I would prefer that you stay here with us, but when you behave that way you'll have to stay by yourself" are useful to reinforce this feeling.

USING THE
TELEPHONE

COMMON
COMPLAINTS

MINOR
INFECTIONS

INFECTIOUS
DISEASES

EMERGENCY
PROBLEMS

NEW INFANT
CARE

PEDIATRIC
PROBLEMS

When your child is being punished, the punishment should be presented in a firm, forceful manner. This is especially important for younger children, who learn best by having the punishment follow *immediately* after they have done something wrong. If you believe that a discussion detailing the reasons for the punishment is necessary, save it for later in the day. Some children have the ability to argue their case with the agility of a good lawyer, and a long discussion at the time of the incident will often make it difficult to teach an important lesson. For those few times when your child convinces you during the *later* discussion that he was right and you were wrong, apologize for your mistake but do not let it deter you from punishing your child the next time it is appropriate.

6. *Be consistent with discipline:* When you discipline your child, punishments should be predictable so that your child can avoid them. It is not nearly as important for a household to be either strict or liberal as it is for the parents to be consistent about those things a child is allowed to do or not do. Many children feel especially insecure when they are not certain of the boundaries to their behavior. They will constantly test their parents to determine where those boundaries are.

7. *Reward normal behavior:* It is a common mistake for many parents who believe that their children have discipline problems to give them much more attention for acting poorly than they do when their youngsters are well behaved. If you discipline your child for acting poorly at the table, but say only to yourself "Thank goodness Johnny acted well today," it is to his advantage to do things you find unpleasant. When it is necessary to punish your children, you should show as little emotion as possible so that your children will get little attention during this time. However, when they behave normally or do something especially well, the praise you give should be enthusiastic, so that your child understands that this is behavior that will be properly rewarded.

Summary

Most problems of behavior can be helped by isolating the problems and applying rewards, punishments and changes in environment in a consistent way. When you discover that your child's problem is at home, school, or with friends, unless it is particularly severe, simple guidance may be all that is necessary. If two of these three areas are affected, you should seek professional counseling early. When all three areas are affected, get help at once since your child has no place to take refuge from his problems.

EATING PROBLEMS
(TOO MUCH OR TOO LITTLE)

Children's eating habits are strongly influenced by their parents' feelings. These are based on culture, past experience, concerns about health, pressure from other family members, and personality. Fears about children not eating enough food usually begin when the child is approximately one-and-one-half years of age. During the first year, children gain about fifteen pounds (a 300 percent increase in weight) but gain only about five pounds during the second year (a 20 percent increase in weight). For this reason, their eating habits change dramatically until about the age of four. Many children begin to eat only one good meal per day at about a year of age, in addition to small snacks taken at regular intervals.

Because parents believe their children are not eating enough, they may begin feeding them cookies and other snack foods with the rationalization that "at least he's eating something". This is a very harmful practice, since in addition to teaching these children to eat junk food, they are also being taught to overeat.

As the child becomes older, parents will often warn, "You can't get up from the table until you finish everything on your plate." Complaints that "I'm full" or "I'm not hungry" are ignored. Worst of all, the child is then rewarded for overeating when his parent says, "You're a good boy. Now I'll give you dessert." It is no wonder that as adults they find themselves overfilling their stomachs at mealtime and then rewarding themselves with dessert.

Those parents who use food as a reward for good behavior are providing their children with a similar disservice. "If you're a good boy I'll give you a cookie," has the obvious effect of equating food with love. A child who feels insecure may then look for food as a way of relieving feelings of anxiety, and may carry this behavior into his adult years.

Other factors that contribute to "fattening up" children include the silly rationale that cookies and milk make a good afternoon snack. When asked why a 3 o'clock small meal is not offered, parents reply that they don't want their child to lose his appetite for dinner. Also, the idea that small children have not eaten enough when they did not finish a portion that was adult-sized is far from realistic.

The inability to help overweight children slim down is one of the major failures of modern medicine. Putting overweight children on a diet *against their will* is virtually impossible, and many doctors believe that it is probably not worth the effort. After the fighting, discussions, and

USING THE TELEPHONE

COMMON COMPLAINTS

MINOR INFECTIONS

INFECTIOUS DISEASES

EMERGENCY PROBLEMS

NEW INFANT CARE

PEDIATRIC PROBLEMS

169

USING THE TELEPHONE

COMMON COMPLAINTS

MINOR INFECTIONS

INFECTIOUS DISEASES

EMERGENCY PROBLEMS

NEW INFANT CARE

PEDIATRIC PROBLEMS

infliction of guilt, the small amount of weight which is eventually lost (and usually shortly regained) is of minimal health significance.

When the child (not just the parent) is motivated and requests help to lose weight, the following recommendations may prove helpful:

1. Don't bring junk food into the house. Expecting the children to avoid it when it is available is not fair and places an unnecessary burden on the child.
2. When snacks are required, use regular food. Half a tuna fish sandwich is preferred to pastry or ice cream.
3. At the start, decreasing portions is usually an easier way of decreasing caloric intake than getting a child used to eating different, less fattening foods. Serving a single-meal portion without having a platter of food on the table to tempt him to take "doubles" is also helpful.
4. Food should be eaten only at the table and placed on a plate. It is easy to lose track of how much you are eating when doing -homework and watching TV. When food is eaten from a container or a box, many children find it difficult to stop until it is all finished.
5. Try to make the diet as small an issue in the home as possible. It should be treated in a matter-of-fact manner with the expectation that the youngster will succeed.
6. Encourage your child to increase his exercise level from whatever is normally done. Walking or bicycle riding may be suggested to non-athletes.

There are true metabolic differences between one child and another. With similar exercise levels and calorie intakes, one child may still be thin while the other may be fat. In addition, some children who do not overeat may be thought to be overweight when, in fact, they simply have a different body shape.

When trying to determine what your child's ideal weight should be, you may use standard height-weight charts as a guide, but they are often inaccurate for any one particular child. Children tend to inherit their fat distribution and bony frames. A wide, stocky child should obviously weigh more than one who has a slight, narrow build. When your child is undressed, if he looks too fat, he most likely is.

You have a responsibility to help him lose weight if he is truly obese and unhappy about it. If he feels no psychological or physical stress about being overweight, apply only minimal pressure as an incentive toward dieting, since all that results from too much pushing is a lot of family fighting and not much else.

When you believe that your child is a *poor eater*, looking at him objectively is a real help. If he looks well nourished, he is probably eating enough, unless he is being fed large amounts of sweets. Contrary to common belief, vitamin supplements do not stimulate appetite, and while they may be offered to a child with erratic eating habits, they are not a substitute for good nutrition.

Periodically, offer your child foods that are of good quality but that you may not enjoy yourself. One parent may enjoy carrots, peas, and string beans and dislike Brussels sprouts, cauliflower, and asparagus, while another parent's tastes may be the reverse. The disliked foods are often not brought home for the child because they aren't even considered. The child, however, may find these to be much more to his liking, and wonder why his parents were so silly as not to feed them to him sooner.

If you honestly believe your child to be poorly nourished or grossly overweight, arrange to discuss these problems with his doctor.

USING THE TELEPHONE

COMMON COMPLAINTS

MINOR INFECTIONS

INFECTIOUS DISEASES

EMERGENCY PROBLEMS

NEW INFANT CARE

PEDIATRIC PROBLEMS

171

USING THE TELEPHONE

COMMON COMPLAINTS

MINOR INFECTIONS

INFECTIOUS DISEASES

EMERGENCY PROBLEMS

NEW INFANT CARE

PEDIATRIC PROBLEMS

SLEEPING PROBLEMS

Since eating, sleeping, and going to the bathroom are basic functions, "sleeping problems" are a frequent cause of concern to parents. However, parents often admit that their real worry isn't that a lack of sleep is going to be dangerous to their child's health. The real problem is that the youngster who sleeps poorly may cause damage to the *parents'* mental and physical health. This is reflected in such remarks as "I need him to take a nap" or "Getting him to sleep at night is so difficult that it is absolutely driving me crazy."

In order to deal with childhood "sleeping problems," we must examine the sleeping patterns of small children. Most children do in fact require more sleep than adults. The reason for this is not certain, although it has been suggested that in terms of evolution, if we were living in the wild, a small defenseless infant would be less likely to be discovered and harmed if he were lying quietly.* (The same would be true for those who are ill or elderly.)

Infants

Because newborn infants require so much food, it is necessary for them to awaken to eat at three- to four-hour intervals. Many parents treat their infant's middle-of-the-night feedings as one of the major disadvantages of having a new baby. Elaborate schemes, long discussions, juggling of diet, and a variety of maneuvers are instituted to get the baby to sleep through the night. Despite these tricks, most babies persist in their efforts to get food until their major growth spurt is nearly completed (at approximately two to three months). Some infants will sleep through the night as early as two weeks after birth, but there are just as many who will not sleep all night until they are four or five months old. Ten to twelve weeks is the average.

In addition to satisfying the infant's protest at not being fed, middle-of-the-night feedings serve another purpose. It is one of the few times during the day when the parent has virtually no distractions and can pay complete attention to the baby. This early bonding is especially impor-

*Carl Sagan, *Dragons of Eden* (New York: Random House, 1977).

172

tant for second and third children, when a hectic daytime schedule will not allow the same luxury of time one has during the rearing of the first child.

Toddlers

When children begin their second year and their rate of growth decreases twelve-fold, their sleep requirements decrease from approximately twelve–fourteen hours to ten–twelve hours per day. Very few youngsters will sleep more than ten hours at night and those that do often will not require a daytime nap. During this period some mothers complain that they can't get the children to bed at night when in fact they are sleeping from 10:00 P.M. to 8:00 A.M. and taking two one-hour naps during the day. The frustration of not being able to eat a quiet dinner or have a casual conversation with a spouse can sometimes be overwhelming and can give the feeling that the day "will never end."

The second group of parents includes those whose children sleep from 8:00 P.M. to 6:00 A.M. and who find getting up so early unpleasant. Those children who sleep from 8:00 P.M. to 8:00 A.M. have parents from the third group who are distraught because their child won't take a nap.

Much of the anxiety comes from the realization that taking care of small children is a very hard job. As with other projects that are worthwhile, long, hard hours are required and sometimes the worker needs a reprieve. Anxiety also comes as a result of not being realistic about the child's true sleeping pattern. Putting the child to sleep two hours before his real bedtime only results in two hours of cuddling, coaxing, feeding, crying (both by the child and the parent), and lots of frustration. If he were put to bed at his real bedtime, the evenings would still be difficult, but they would be much more pleasant.

If adjustments are going to be made to induce a child to go to sleep earlier or to nap in the afternoon, one must start during the morning hours. That is, wake the child up a few hours earlier if you are attempting to change his schedule.

Bedtime is a very stressful experience for many young children. It is their first consistent exposure to separation from their parents. Their fear may be expressed as repeated requests for a bottle (don't give it unless you don't mind rotten teeth), juice, a cookie, one more hug, or a lost doll. The child may "just want to tell you something," want you to "make that weird shadow go away," and suddenly remember "something I have to do now" or that "I forgot to go to the bathroom."

Through this barrage of requests, be sympathetic and forceful at the same time. "I know you feel scared of monsters and I honestly feel badly

173

USING THE TELEPHONE

COMMON COMPLAINTS

MINOR INFECTIONS

INFECTIOUS DISEASES

EMERGENCY PROBLEMS

NEW INFANT CARE

PEDIATRIC PROBLEMS

USING THE TELEPHONE

COMMON COMPLAINTS

MINOR INFECTIONS

INFECTIOUS DISEASES

EMERGENCY PROBLEMS

NEW INFANT CARE

PEDIATRIC PROBLEMS

for you, but monsters aren't allowed in our house and now you must go to bed." Talking about pleasant things is also a reasonable distraction. Assuming that there aren't any major emotional problems, younger children should be allowed to cry themselves to sleep on occasion. It may take no more than three nights to change a child's schedule, and this method has much less potential for causing psychological trauma than a chronically overtired parent will during daytime hours. Sedatives should be avoided unless there is a specific medical reason for them. Discuss them with your physician before using them.

Cribs

Different parents choose different ages at which to move their children from a crib into a bed. Generally, if your child can climb over the crib rails, he should be moved into a bed to prevent a middle-of-the-night injury. If you are concerned about your child hurting himself by wandering about the house while you are sleeping, one eyelet may be screwed into the door and one into the doorframe. Join them with a piece of string in such a way that the child may open the door a few inches to call out for help but cannot get through without attracting attention.

Another appropriate time to move your youngster into a bed is when you have made the transition to thinking of him as a thinking person and not as a baby. When he is verbal, in a play group, and interacting at a more advanced social level with you, sleeping in a crib may no longer be appropriate.

Sleep Requirements

Sleep requirements vary not only by age group but also on an individual basis. Some children simply require more or less sleep than others. If your child sleeps six hours a night and wakes up appearing fresh when leaving for school, he probably does not need more sleep. Because sleep requirements may be hereditary, a true family conflict may arise if the mother requires an extra amount of sleep, and the father and children do not. This inequality of sleep needs may give the appearance of a mother who is nervous, depressed, tired, and ill when all she needs is two more hours of sleep at night. While this biological variation cannot be changed, having an awareness of these differences may be of tremendous help in solving some otherwise difficult family problems.

174

TOILET TRAINING

Although most children are physically ready to be toilet-trained when their coordination allows them to run well (approximately eighteen to twenty months), most children are not psychologically ready at this time. If your child tells you that she has soiled her pants and wishes to be changed—especially if she does so the same time every day—you may wish to consider toilet training at this time. The majority of children are not truly ready to be toilet-trained until they are approximately two-and-one-half years of age because it is at this time that they can understand cause-and-effect suggestions ("If you do this, that will happen.") If you decide to begin toilet training your child before two-and-one-half years of age, you should expect her to become "untrained" after being trained. This tends to happen repeatedly and parents should not take each regression as though it were a major setback or personal affront.

A potty chair that sits on the floor should be used in preference to a training seat that snaps onto an adult toilet seat. The potty chair is preferred because the child can go to the toilet without help from her parents and because allowing her feet to touch the ground will make it much easier for her to pass a hard bowel movement.

You should try to choose a time to make your child familiar with the potty chair when you are not hurried and when there is little chance of your being called away. Reading materials for you to look at together are helpful and this training time should be treated as a regular part of your child's day. Once your child is willing to sit on the seat (with or without a diaper) training should begin in earnest.

Whenever your child soils a diaper, you should let her know that you are unhappy with what she did, but give her very little attention for doing so. In an unemotional way you should tell her that "I don't want you to go in your diaper anymore. Now you are supposed to use the potty." If your child learns that you get upset when she soils a diaper, it will be only a short time before she learns to use this technique to get your attention whenever she wishes it. Also, because your child will initially soil a diaper more frequently than she will use the potty, you will be giving her much more attention for doing the wrong thing than the right thing as the weeks progress.

When your child does go to the bathroom in the proper place, you should be very encouraging to her, using hugging, kissing, and clapping. Charts with stars or other similar devices may be very useful. It is advisable not to use food or toys as rewards for toilet training.

175

USING THE TELEPHONE

COMMON COMPLAINTS

MINOR INFECTIONS

INFECTIOUS DISEASES

EMERGENCY PROBLEMS

NEW INFANT CARE

PEDIATRIC PROBLEMS

USING THE TELEPHONE

COMMON COMPLAINTS

MINOR INFECTIONS

INFECTIOUS DISEASES

EMERGENCY PROBLEMS

NEW INFANT CARE

PEDIATRIC PROBLEMS

In summary, using a potty chair is preferable to using a trainer seat for toilet training. Do not train your child before she is psychologically ready. Also do not be discouraged if training takes a long time or if your youngster has frequent setbacks during the early training period. Give your child as little attention as possible when she soils her diaper, but be very enthusiastic when she achieves her goal.

BED-WETTING
(ENURESIS)

Bed-wetting should not be considered a problem unless your child is older than six years, since approximately 20 percent of children at age five are still wetting their beds at regular intervals. There is frequently a family tendency toward bed-wetting, and your child is more likely to have this problem if one of his parents was a bed-wetter.

If your child wets frequently during the day or has never had a period when he was dry at night, contact your physician to be certain that there are no medical problems contributing to the bed-wetting. When your child can remain dry during the entire day or if there have been regular periods when he has been dry at night, the chance of there being something wrong with his bladder or kidneys is relatively small.

You can help your child avoid wetting his bed by not allowing him to drink large quantities of fluid after dinner (many children who ask for a drink at bedtime are not really thirsty and will be content just taking sips of juice or milk). Have him go to the toilet just before going to sleep and, during the early stages of night training, you may wish to bring him to the bathroom just before your own bedtime. If these simple methods fail, using a chart that gives your child stars for nights when he has remained dry may be useful. A reward may be used initially for one dry night, then for three dry nights, and later for five dry nights, until longer periods without wetting become more usual. On those nights when your child wets the bed, you should give him as little attention as possible but encourage him to do better the following night.

On some occasions, your physician may wish to prescribe a medicine such as Imipramine to relax the bladder and allow it to hold more urine. This medicine is not usually used for children under six years. Side effects are relatively uncommon. Training devices, such as electric buzzers and lights, should generally be avoided.

Although bed-wetting may have an emotional component in some cases, more often than not these children have no special psychological problems. Nighttime training is easy for many youngsters but can be embarrassing and a source of frustration for many others. Patience and perseverance pay off.

USING THE TELEPHONE

COMMON COMPLAINTS

MINOR INFECTIONS

INFECTIOUS DISEASES

EMERGENCY PROBLEMS

NEW INFANT CARE

PEDIATRIC PROBLEMS

177

USING THE TELEPHONE

COMMON COMPLAINTS

MINOR INFECTIONS

INFECTIOUS DISEASES

EMERGENCY PROBLEMS

NEW INFANT CARE

PEDIATRIC PROBLEMS

THE "SPOILED" CHILD

From infancy, children use many techniques for controlling their parents. They begin by using two very distinct cries. The first type of cry is loud, shrill, and piercing, and is especially effective at two in the morning. This intimidating cry is used in much the same way that parents intimidate their children by yelling at them. The second type of cry has a pathetic, whimpering quality that effectively makes parents feel guilty if they don't respond. In addition, as the infant becomes older and begins to socialize, he learns the more sophisticated technique of rewarding his parents with a smile or hug when the parent has done something nice for him.

This early communication of the need for attention is especially effective for first children, whose parents have a tendency to stop what they are doing to pick baby up at its first "peep." By the time the second and third children have arrived, the parents have usually learned to finish what they were doing before responding to the baby.

Being "spoiled" is a relative term. Conservative parents will refer to a demanding child as being spoiled while liberal parents may refer to him as being "very willful." It is difficult for us to make a formal definition, except that we are discussing children here who expect others to do things for them that they should do themselves, and who are very intolerant when others do not respond quickly to their demands. Appropriate behavior for a younger child is obviously not appropriate for an older one, and spoiled children will occasionally be referred to as babyish.

When trying to decide if your child is spoiled, you must first develop a reasonable expectation of normal behavior for your child's age group. As we have discussed above, most children begin by being demanding and self-centered and only gradually learn that others around them are important also. Parents who are afraid to set *reasonable* limits to their child's behavior because they are afraid that the child won't love them frequently have the opposite happen. Children who are not given boundaries may feel very insecure because they do not yet understand the world around them. However, do not be angry with your child for trying to ignore these limits. If he were totally compliant it would mean that he wasn't looking out for *his* best interests and would eventually suffer for it.

When possible, both parents should set the specific limits. Being strict or not strict is not nearly as important as being consistent and predictable. Also, these limits should not be hypocritical in terms of the rela-

178

tive demands that parents make on themselves. When your children become young adults and are not under constant supervision, they may not make the same decisions you would have made when confronted with a difficult situation, but they should have a reasonably good idea of what you would have chosen. They will then give that choice strong consideration if they respect you.

USING THE
TELEPHONE

COMMON
COMPLAINTS

MINOR
INFECTIONS

INFECTIOUS
DISEASES

EMERGENCY
PROBLEMS

NEW INFANT
CARE

PEDIATRIC
PROBLEMS

USING THE TELEPHONE

COMMON COMPLAINTS

MINOR INFECTIONS

INFECTIOUS DISEASES

EMERGENCY PROBLEMS

NEW INFANT CARE

PEDIATRIC PROBLEMS

FEARFULNESS

Children of many ages become fearful of different things and at different times of the day. Two- to three-year-olds will be especially upset at bedtime and complain about moving shadows, monsters, and darkness (see "Sleeping Problems"). However, parents will express special concern about their child's personality or adjustment when he seems to become "afraid of everything." It is true that children who have periods of extreme fearfulness may have underlying psychological problems, or there may be real or imagined incidents that cause them to become especially upset. However, fearfulness should be considered part of the normal developing process.

When children are toddlers, they are usually not afraid of anything and parents must use constant supervision to assure their safety. After a period of experimenting and learning, children eventually realize that certain actions and things may be dangerous and harmful to them. Once they learn that they really *can* be harmed, they may find it difficult to sort out those things which won't harm them from those which will. It is during this time that periods of fearfulness develop.

Tell your child that being afraid can actually be a good thing because it keeps us from being harmed, and that he should trust you to tell him which things aren't dangerous. Most important, be sympathetic in your feelings but firm in your statements as you are being reassuring. "I know that you feel afraid of the darkness. Everyone feels that way sometimes, but we absolutely will not allow anything to hurt you while you are asleep."

SHYNESS

It is a frequent mistake for parents to believe that childhood is almost always a fun experience without the frustrations and anxieties that are present in adult life. One has only to reflect on being called to answer a question in school and standing red-faced and sweating in front of the class to remember one of many childhood anxieties.

Although children's personalities can obviously be influenced by their self-confidence, environment, and past experience, they also have temperaments similar to those of adults. At a party consisting of ten "grown-ups," we will usually find two who are outgoing and introduce themselves with a firm voice and handshake. Another two will be shy and tend to stand off by themselves, trying to hide their uneasiness. The remaining six will begin by feeling shy but will gradually become more social once conversation gets started.

Children tend to follow the same patterns in their personalities. Often, a child's personality is not very different from those of her parents. Shy parents may be most upset when their children appear shy because they do not want them to suffer the same social unease they themselves have felt.

Remember that not all children are outgoing, happy, and social toward each other. To a reasonable degree, shyness is perfectly normal. If your child has a tendency to be shy, don't say she's "silly for being that way" but explain that you understand how she feels and that "everyone feels shy but some people are better at hiding their feelings than others." Ease her slowly but firmly into difficult social situations, and be reassuring about her ability to succeed despite nervousness.

After the age of four, if shyness becomes so extreme that your child cannot socialize with other children, consult your physician or a trained professional.

USING THE TELEPHONE

COMMON COMPLAINTS

MINOR INFECTIONS

INFECTIOUS DISEASES

EMERGENCY PROBLEMS

NEW INFANT CARE

PEDIATRIC PROBLEMS

USING THE TELEPHONE

COMMON COMPLAINTS

MINOR INFECTIONS

INFECTIOUS DISEASES

EMERGENCY PROBLEMS

NEW INFANT CARE

PEDIATRIC PROBLEMS

THE MIDDLE CHILD

Those parents who don't believe that their child will enter the "terrible twos" are just as surprised when they find that their middle child has the "middle-child syndrome." These children have the problem position of not being allowed to copy the first child ("You're not old enough to do that") and not being allowed to get attention for being babyish ("You're not a baby anymore. You are not allowed to do that"). This middle position is not improved when the first two children are close in age and the third is born long afterward, since the oldest child remains the oldest but the second child has been displaced and is no longer the "baby."

If your child has been caught in this middle role, help him to find a place for himself rather than put emphasis on his being well rounded. If you see that your child has an interest in sports, music, art, or language skills, encourage participation in those activities that will strengthen these aptitudes so he will develop a talent that will help him to feel secure. Do not push this single activity to the exclusion of all others, but emphasize it whenever possible. Tell your middle child that you understand his plight and that you will help him through it, but don't allow him to take advantage of your "understanding" to the degree that he does not have to perform appropriately.

THE HYPERACTIVE CHILD
(MINIMAL BRAIN DYSFUNCTION, ATTENTION-DEFICIT DISORDER)

Children are referred to as hyperactive or hyperkinetic when they are more active than others of their age group. Since there is a full spectrum of activity among children, this judgment is a relative one. Our discussion here refers to those children who have a short attention span and difficulty sitting still or concentrating on their work, and are thought by their parents and/or their teachers to have a behavior problem. They may also have some minor neurologic difficulties, such as eye-hand incoordination, clumsiness, and/or learning disability. Because this "hyperactive syndrome" has been popularized in recent years, children who have difficulty with behavior and are not "doing well in school" may have been classified as being hyperactive by teachers as a means of shifting the blame for poor performance from the school to the child. However, there are children who clearly fit the strict criteria outlined above and who profit from proper evaluation.

Oftentimes, parents and teachers are first strict, then lenient, and then strict again with a hyperactive child. Because these children are singled out as being a nuisance, many of them will also develop psychological problems from not knowing what the acceptable boundaries of behavior are. They then develop a poor self-image in addition to their initial problem of hyperactivity.

Children who are unable to concentrate—those who are hyperactive and those who are not—are frequently referred to as "daydreamers." Because of this inability to concentrate both of these groups have been classified as having an *attention-deficit disorder* (A.D.D.).

The following information may be useful to parents who believe that their child is hyperactive:

1. There are two major causes of hyperactivity:
   a. *Emotional problems* alone may cause nervousness or an inability to concentrate that may be confused with a true hyperactivity syndrome. To treat this group of youngsters, one must determine the source of their anxiety and deal with it appropriately.
   b. The group described as having "minimal brain dysfunction" or "minimal brain damage" (M.B.D.) have a *neurologic* inability to concentrate and may become hyperactive because they cannot keep their minds on track. This may be the result of birth trauma, a hereditary trait (the parents were also hyperactive), a major neuro-

USING THE TELEPHONE

COMMON COMPLAINTS

MINOR INFECTIONS

INFECTIOUS DISEASES

EMERGENCY PROBLEMS

NEW INFANT CARE

PEDIATRIC PROBLEMS

183

USING THE
TELEPHONE

COMMON
COMPLAINTS

MINOR
INFECTIONS

INFECTIOUS
DISEASES

EMERGENCY
PROBLEMS

NEW INFANT
CARE

PEDIATRIC
PROBLEMS

logic problem including a seizure disorder (this is less common), or an allergy or reaction to a food or food additive. The role of diet, especially food colorings and naturally occurring salicylates (the active ingredient in aspirin), is controversial but certainly it affects at least a small percentage of these children.

2. *Diagnosis*

There are *no specific diagnostic tests* for the hyperactive child syndrome. The diagnosis should be made by a pediatrician, psychologist, and neurologist; the latter two should be dealing with children on a regular basis. This diagnosis is made as much by reviewing the child's history thoroughly as by performing a complete physical examination. Symptoms are often present from infancy. Many of these children were irritable, cranky, or colicky and had difficulty accepting affection.

It is useful to note that the hyperactivity associated with this neurologic syndrome has a "searching" or flowing quality while the hyperactivity seen with anxiety or nervousness may have a more repetitive "foot-tapping" or "finger-drumming" quality.

3. *Treatment*

Because a small percentage of these children may have *diet-related* symptoms, many pediatricians suggest that the diet proposed by Dr. Benjamin Feingold be given a trial. The diet is quite difficult to maintain properly and may be obtained by purchasing Dr. Feingold's books or by consulting with your pediatrician. Some children may also have a very obvious change in personality when foods containing concentrated sweets, caffeine (coffee, tea, cola), and chocolate (chocolate is similar biochemically to caffeine) are avoided. Aside from the stimulant or sedative effect of caffeine, frequent swings of blood sugar throughout the day may definitely influence the temperament of some children. Laboratory tests, such as a five-hour glucose tolerance test, are sometimes used for the diagnosis of susceptible children, but they are painful, expensive, and not nearly as reliable as simply changing your child's diet. Moreover, avoiding these foods is generally in your child's best interest since foods with poor nutritional value are being excluded. Caffeine can be avoided by noting it in the ingredients of a food's label. Foods which list sugar or forms of sugar (sucrose, dextrose, molasses, etcetera) as one of the first three ingredients should also be avoided.

Establishing a structured environment for the child to help her find boundaries while giving appropriate rewards for good behavior are necessary for both the child and her parents. Help from a counselor may be necessary for this part of treatment. See the introductory section of this chapter.

Medicines that help to increase attention span have unequivocally been shown to be useful for the majority of children with attention-deficit disorder. Parents will often express the fear that these medicines are addicting and that they will be "drugging their child into submission" because they act as stimulants for adults. Generally your physician will not prescribe these very useful medicines unless your child is having great difficulty functioning on a daily basis. When this occurs, your child is taking a specific medicine for a specific neurologic disorder in much the same way that a patient with asthma may need medications to avoid wheezing on a regular basis. Side effects from these medicines, when taken in proper dosage, are minimal. The benefits to your child may be major, helping her to concentrate on schoolwork, and improving behavior to the point where the people around her may be able to relate to her in a much more normal way.

4. *Outcome (prognosis)*

Many children with an attention-deficit disorder and hyperactivity seem to show a general improvement as they approach their adolescent years, but much of their future will depend on how well they have adjusted their personalities to their underlying neurologic problem. A poorly adjusted adult who is hyperactive is thought of as a nuisance, a boor, or a troublemaker. However, adults with this syndrome will be referred to as go-getters and successfully aggressive when their hyperactivity is channeled into socially acceptable projects. Poorly adjusted adults with an attention-deficit disorder who are not hyperactive will be referred to as spacy, airheads, or flaky, but those who have compensated for their condition will appear calm, stable, and a little absentminded.

For these reasons, the attention-deficit disorder should be examined aggressively by parents and therapists, especially when it is obvious that the child is dealing with her handicap poorly.

USING THE TELEPHONE

COMMON COMPLAINTS

MINOR INFECTIONS

INFECTIOUS DISEASES

EMERGENCY PROBLEMS

NEW INFANT CARE

PEDIATRIC PROBLEMS

USING THE
TELEPHONE

COMMON
COMPLAINTS

MINOR
INFECTIONS

INFECTIOUS
DISEASES

EMERGENCY
PROBLEMS

NEW INFANT
CARE

PEDIATRIC
PROBLEMS

NON-NERVOUS "NERVOUS" HABITS

These conditions are referred to here as non-nervous "nervous" habits because although they may be *aggravated* by nervousness, they are not *caused* by nervousness. Many of these children are not more nervous than their peers, but have symptoms which develop during stresses which are faced by all children.

Tics or Mannerisms

Frequent and spontaneous mannerisms, also called twitches or tics (usually of the face but which may affect any body part), can occur at any age but most often begin between ages seven and ten. In the past, they were thought to be related to excessive nervousness but are now believed to be an expression of an increased irritation to the nervous system. It is not unusual for these youngsters to have at least one parent who also has the disorder, indicating that there may be a hereditary component. These "tics" become worse when the child is overtired, under stress or nervous, or is being bothered by an illness or allergies.

Because they may affect the eyes, parents will frequently see an eye specialist for advice despite the absence of a true eye abnormality. However, if your child is constantly squinting, nearsightedness should be suspected. When facial tics and voice tics (making sounds involuntarily) occur together, discuss them with your doctor.

Treatment consists of correcting as many of the underlying irritating factors as possible. Ensuring adequate rest, removing allergy-causing agents, and trying to avoid stressful situations will all be helpful. The child should be told that the "tic" is not his fault. Tell him that you realize other children may sometimes make fun of it when they notice it, and that this may cause him to feel embarrassed or ashamed, but that real friends will certainly not make fun of him.

Generally, such children should be treated as though they have a *cosmetic* problem rather than a *nervous* condition. Be sympathetic to their concerns without giving them undue attention. The more upset you become, the more self-conscious your child will feel.

186

The problem may disappear for long periods of time only to recur at a later age. Do not feel that these recurrences are a major setback since they should be expected.

Medicines have been used experimentally. Most have unpleasant side effects and are not generally used unless the child is badly bothered by the disorder.

Stuttering

This condition tends to have some family predisposition and may be worse during periods of stress. It should also not be thought of as a "nervous" problem, although the stuttering may have a tendency to *make* the child feel nervous.

Many children between the ages of two and four have a temporary period of stuttering as they attempt to rush their thoughts into speech. The stutter may worsen if parents pressure the child with statements such as "slow down and start again." For this reason, and because the condition usually disappears by itself, parents are frequently told to ignore the child's speech problem. The difficulty with this approach is that the child wonders why her parents are so foolish as not to notice her frustration at not being able to "get her words out." It is more reasonable therefore for the parent to stop what he is doing when the child is talking (when practical) and to face the child during conversations. He should also be empathetic with her problems by discussing them with her in a way that does not put pressure on her. As an example, you might wish to say, "I know that it is difficult for you to get the words out and it may sometimes get you upset. You will see that it will become easier for you soon."

Try not to let your child see your anxiety at her stuttering. If you believe that the condition is worsening rather than improving or if there is a family history of major speech problems, discuss this matter with your physician.

USING THE TELEPHONE

COMMON COMPLAINTS

MINOR INFECTIONS

INFECTIOUS DISEASES

EMERGENCY PROBLEMS

NEW INFANT CARE

PEDIATRIC PROBLEMS

USING THE
TELEPHONE

COMMON
COMPLAINTS

MINOR
INFECTIONS

INFECTIOUS
DISEASES

EMERGENCY
PROBLEMS

NEW INFANT
CARE

NERVOUS HABITS

Thumbsucking and Nailbiting

These habits have been grouped together because they are voluntary as distinguished from tics, which cannot be controlled by the child. Both of these are exaggerated during times when the child is nervous or upset but the presence of nailbiting or thumbsucking does not necessarily mean that your youngster is a "nervous child."

It is difficult to effectively help your child to stop these habits before the age of four. A type of behavior modification similar to that used for toilet training or bed-wetting is the most successful approach. Your child should be rewarded for *not* thumbsucking or nailbiting during periods of time he can master relatively easily. Charts to be filled with stars or boxes filled in with colored markers that lead to a prize when completed are useful. Larger rewards should be given when longer periods of time are achieved: first for mealtimes, then for whole morning or afternoon sessions, and lastly for the most difficult period—bedtime. When the child succeeds he should be highly praised. When he fails he should be encouraged to do better next time with as little discussion as possible. Children who appear "cured" will frequently revert to their habits in much the same way that adult cigarette smokers do, but these relapses should not be treated as though your child has committed a terrible act. Rather, he should be encouraged to try to stop once again using the techniques outlined above as frequently as is necessary.

PROBLEMS OF WORKING MOTHERS

Because of social trends and financial pressures many mothers with young children have returned to paying jobs. Those who return to work have had a difficult decision to make as they try to balance their desire to be home with their children with feelings of wanting to bring home money or enter a more stimulating environment. When the family financial situation makes it necessary to return to work or if a mother is able to obtain a part-time job, the decision is somewhat easier. However, when the mother is free to choose, the situation that makes her feel the *least guilty*, rather than the one she *prefers* the most, is most likely to reflect her true feelings.

If a mother is at work and spends much of her day feeling guilty that she is not at home with her child, then she probably should be at home. On the other hand, when mothers who are at home resent their children for hindering their careers or not allowing them to fulfill other needs which they believe are more important, they would most likely be more content at a paying job. What is right for one mother may not be right for someone else, and what is proper for you might prove to be a terribly wrong decision for your friend.

Disregard decisions that were made before the baby was born until you are actually at home in the mothering role. We have talked with many mothers who intended to return to work after two or three weeks only to find that despite a strong career interest, they really wanted to remain at home with their small infants. Other mothers believed that the chores of motherhood would be fun and later came to think of them as boring and couldn't wait to return to work. These decisions are certainly not easy, but your child will benefit most if you are honest about the decision that makes you feel the least guilty.

USING THE TELEPHONE

COMMON COMPLAINTS

MINOR INFECTIONS

INFECTIOUS DISEASES

EMERGENCY PROBLEMS

NEW INFANT CARE

PEDIATRIC PROBLEMS

SEX EDUCATION

Parents frequently call pediatricians to ask them for books or literature relating to reproduction, menstruation, and other similar topics. When choosing a book to help you instruct your children, choose one with which you feel comfortable. A reference discussing sex in a matter-of-fact, simplistic way might be perfectly appropriate in a home where sexual matters would not normally be considered as regular conversation, but would be totally inappropriate in a liberal household where sexual matters are discussed openly. An explicitly diagrammed manual, on the other hand, might be proper in the second home but would be totally out of place in the first.

In discussing sexual matters with your child, use terms which are easy for you to deal with rather than those that someone told you were right or wrong. Giving your explanation in a relaxed manner without giving the impression that sex is dirty, naughty, or mystical is more important than using someone else's words. You may find it useful to read one or two books for information concerning the topics you are discussing, even though you may feel that those books are not appropriate for your youngsters.

Menstruation:

Since sex education has become more common in grade schools, there are fewer situations in which physicians are requested to discuss menstruation with girls. When discussing menstruation with your daughter, review the material that she was taught in school since her teacher may not have been especially knowledgeable. The following information may be useful to her:

1. Her menstrual period may not come every twenty-eight days during the first year. They are often not regular at first and should be considered normal even if they come at odd times.
2. Most girls do not have painful menstruation. Some youngsters may be fooled into thinking that everyone has pain during her menstrual period because only those girls with cramps discuss them, while those who have no symptoms do not complain. In most cases, the first few years of menstruation are not accompanied by cramping because they are not associated with making ova or eggs.

3. It is not necessary to wait before using tampons. The use or non-use of tampons as opposed to pads is a personal matter but there is a common misconception that menstruating teenagers must wait at least one or two years before they can be inserted. There is no medical reason why they cannot be used early. Many girls, however, prefer to use pads initially so that they can observe menstrual flow while it is an unfamiliar experience.

If tampons are preferred, you should tell your daughter: (a) to buy a variety of different brands so that she might choose a shape and applicator that she will feel comfortable with; (b) she should attempt to insert the tampon at a time when she is not menstruating so that she will not have to worry that improper insertion might cause her embarrassment. A lubricant such as Vaseline may be helpful during initial insertions; (c) she should avoid using tampons containing deodorants since they may be irritating; (d) tampons should not be used during the entire menstrual cycle because, although the "toxic shock syndrome" (fever, vomiting, rash leading to shock) is very uncommon, the chances of getting an infection surrounding the tampon may be decreased significantly by alternating tampons with pads. Many girls prefer to use tampons during the day so as not to restrict their activity and to use pads at night when they are sleeping. High-absorbency tampons also appear to carry greater risk than less absorbent types that must be changed more frequently.

USING THE TELEPHONE

COMMON COMPLAINTS

MINOR INFECTIONS

INFECTIOUS DISEASES

EMERGENCY PROBLEMS

NEW INFANT CARE

PEDIATRIC PROBLEMS

191

USING THE TELEPHONE

COMMON COMPLAINTS

MINOR INFECTIONS

INFECTIOUS DISEASES

EMERGENCY PROBLEMS

NEW INFANT CARE

PEDIATRIC PROBLEMS

SEPARATION, DIVORCE AND YOUR CHILD

When parents have decided to live separately, the children who are involved may receive only part of the attention they deserve. Both parents have lawyers (and often therapists) who specifically act as advocates for *them*, but there is usually no one specifically to look after the children's interests. If your physician feels comfortable in this role of child advocate, he will request a meeting with both parents to offer suggestions for dealing with the children's anxieties. If he personally would prefer not to counsel parents, he is usually a good source for an appropriate referral.

Regardless of the circumstances of the separation or divorce, most children who are involved in these confrontations have similar fears and concerns:

1. Fear of abandonment.
The idea of parents not living together is usually difficult for children to accept. If one parent is leaving home, "How do I know," wonders the child, "that my other parent will not leave me also?" The parent living with the child may not consider it even a remote possibility but the child's perception may be completely different. Even if she does not mention this fear of abandonment, the parent at home should be reassuring in a manner that is not aggressive.

2. Guilt.
Before the actual breakup, tempers are short, patience is limited, and the children may become the objects of parental frustrations. In addition, some youngsters may act out more than usual to gain attention for themselves and also to draw attention away from the parents' fighting. As a result, the child may be left with the impression that the separation occurred because she was acting in a naughty way. Although the child may not express this concern to her parents, she should be reassured that the breakup was not her fault.

3. Fantasy.
No matter how final the separation, children often have a magical feeling that they can bring their parents back together again. Understanding these feelings will put her remarks and actions in greater perspective.

192

Although parents feel many pressures during this time of separation or divorce and may have angry thoughts and feelings, these are some of the ways they can ease their child's discomfort:

(a) *Adding predictability*:

Although it might seem less anxiety-producing to allow casual visiting by the parent who is not living at home, a predictable visiting schedule can change the disappointment of a parent not coming home each night to a workable series of expectations for the child. She will be much more comfortable knowing that her father is coming each Monday and Saturday than she will if her father comes to visit at different times on different weeks.

(b) *Allow your child to discuss her problems*:

When you believe your child to be unhappy, it may be difficult to get yourself to ask if there is anything bothering her. Many children may not offer the information because of their personalities or because they think their parent may not be interested or will become upset. Your child should be asked questions in a manner that does not threaten them or have an accusing tone. "I know something is bothering you. What is it?" will not get the same response as "You have been acting unhappy these past few days. Is there anything that you'd like to talk about?"

Parents themselves may wish not to ask their youngsters these questions simply because they do not want to hear the answers. However, allowing your child to discuss her feelings in her own words is a very important part of helping her adjust to her new situation.

(c) *Avoid messenger tactics*:

Parents should avoid sending messages to each other through their children. During those periods when parents are feeling depressed or upset with the way that their life is going, they may tend to say nasty things about each other, sending negative information to the other parent through the child. Because each parent may try to "better" the other, the children are placed in an extremely difficult role. When a parent receives an inappropriate message through the child, it is extremely important that one parent call the other rather than fall prey to this cruel scheme. Making a simple phone call may require strength and maturity but it is not fair to expect it from your child if you will not do it yourself.

(d) *Allow for communication between parents*:

Regardless of the negative feelings that develop before the breaking up, a regular meeting time should be arranged between

USING THE TELEPHONE

COMMON COMPLAINTS

MINOR INFECTIONS

INFECTIOUS DISEASES

EMERGENCY PROBLEMS

NEW INFANT CARE

PEDIATRIC PROBLEMS

193

USING THE
TELEPHONE

COMMON
COMPLAINTS

MINOR
INFECTIONS

INFECTIOUS
DISEASES

EMERGENCY
PROBLEMS

NEW INFANT
CARE

PEDIATRIC
PROBLEMS

parents at intervals of at least once or twice a year on a strict schedule to discuss nothing other than the children's welfare. Matters concerning health, emotional well-being and school performance, which require a conference between both parents, may not receive proper attention unless specific meeting times have been set aside to discuss them.

(e) *Capitalize on the advantages of separation:*
Separation of parents creates many problems for the children involved. Not living in a home with two incompatible parents may be a major advantage for the child. Allow the children to benefit by involving them in as little future strife as possible.

COPING WITH THE DEATH OF A FAMILY MEMBER OR FRIEND

When a family member or friend has died, you may wish to ask your physician for advice since he will usually be familiar with you and your children. The suggestions he or she gives you will depend on your family practices, the ages of your children, and the circumstances of the death. However, many of the problems which parents face when they are discussing death with children result from not following the advice outlined below:

1. *Be truthful* when discussing with your child what happens after a person dies. If you honestly don't know what happens when someone dies, that is exactly what you should tell your children. If you feel reasonably certain of your beliefs, tell them to your children. Do not tell them something that you don't believe yourself since your children will sense your insincerity and will assume that you are lying because death is so terrible that you cannot tell them what actually happens. It is useful to say, "No one knows for certain what happens after a person dies but we believe that . . ." so that if differing explanations about death are heard from others they might feel more comfortable about the discrepancy.

2. Whenever it is practical, have your children participate in the mourning process along with the family, to the extent that it matches with your individual family practices and customs. Generally, if you would let them be present at a happy event that requires the same discipline from them, they should be allowed to participate here in a similar manner.

Many children feel insecure when they are separated from family members whom they know to be unhappy. Letting them participate in the grieving process reinforces to the children that you think of them as being an active part of the family structure. In addition, the children also may act as a diversion, which gives the rest of the family a feeling of on-goingness during this particularly depressing time.

3. Ask your children about their thoughts and feelings, and be sympathetic with them. If your child feels angry or sad, let him know that these feelings are normal and discuss them with him to help him understand them better.

COMMON COMPLAINTS

MINOR INFECTIONS

INFECTIOUS DISEASES

EMERGENCY PROBLEMS

NEW INFANT CARE

PEDIATRIC PROBLEMS

195

PEDIATRIC
PROBLEMS

NEW INFANT
CARE

EMERGENCY
PROBLEMS

INFECTIOUS
DISEASES

MINOR
INFECTIONS

COMMON
COMPLAINTS

USING THE
TELEPHONE

APPENDIX

Commonly prescribed diets
Clear liquids
Soft-bland
Milk-free

Your doctor's office policy

Your doctor's preferred medicines to relieve symptoms

Consent form for medical treatment

Personal notes

PEDIATRIC PROBLEMS

NEW INFANT CARE

EMERGENCY PROBLEMS

INFECTIOUS DISEASES

MINOR INFECTIONS

COMMON COMPLAINTS

USING THE TELEPHONE

COMMONLY PRESCRIBED DIETS

Clear liquids:

Apple juice
Grape juice
Weak tea with sugar
Flat soda (not diet soda)
Clear soup or bouillon
Jello

Soft-bland diet:

Crackers
Toast with jelly
Applesauce
Banana
Rice or rice cereal
Boiled chicken, eggs, potato

USING THE TELEPHONE

COMMON COMPLAINTS

MINOR INFECTIONS

INFECTIOUS DISEASES

EMERGENCY PROBLEMS

NEW INFANT CARE

PEDIATRIC PROBLEMS

Milk-free diet:

Avoid foods whose labels indicate milk, cheeses, milk products, dry milk, and whey. Always read labels carefully.

Foods to avoid:

Baked goods including rolls (hamburger and hot dog), cookies and breads. Usually OK: Whole wheat bread, rye bread, pumpernickel, hard rolls, and pie crust.

Ice Cream and sherbet. Usually OK: Water or italian ices.

Fried foods, including fish, clams, onion rings, are often dipped in milk before frying. Usually OK: Fried potatoes.

Breaded foods. Bread crumbs are often seasoned with cheese. Stuffing often contains milk. Beware of meatballs. Usually OK: Unseasoned bread crumbs.

Sausage meats, including hot dogs, often have milk products added. Liverwurst, paté may contain large amounts of milk. Usually OK: Kosher meat products.

Candy, especially milk chocolate. Usually OK: Sucking candies and dark chocolate.

Spreads. Some brands of margarine contain milk or whey. Usually OK: All corn oil margarine and butter (which contains only milk fat, not protein or sugar).

Salad dressings frequently contain cheese or cream. Usually OK: Mayonnaise, salad oil.

YOUR DOCTOR'S OFFICE POLICY

(GET THIS INFORMATION FROM THE DOCTOR'S RECEPTIONIST)

Doctor's Name _____

Receptionist's Name _____

Nurse's Name _____

Office Address _____
_____

Regular office hours _____

Weekend and holiday office hours _____

The best route to get to the office _____

Office policy for insurance forms _____
_____

The usual intervals for routine physical exams. _____

How far in advance should they be scheduled? _____

Usual fee schedule. _____
_____

Hospital to go to in case of emergency. _____

Best hour to call the doctor for nonurgent questions. _____

USING THE TELEPHONE

COMMON COMPLAINTS

MINOR INFECTIONS

INFECTIOUS DISEASES

EMERGENCY PROBLEMS

NEW INFANT CARE

PEDIATRIC PROBLEMS

201

USING THE TELEPHONE

COMMON COMPLAINTS

MINOR INFECTIONS

INFECTIOUS DISEASES

EMERGENCY PROBLEMS

NEW INFANT CARE

PEDIATRIC PROBLEMS

YOUR DOCTOR'S PREFERRED MEDICINES TO RELIEVE SYMPTOMS

Child's Name and Age			
Fever			
Stuffy Nose			
Cough			
Earache			
Sore Throat			
Wheezing			
Stomach Cramps			
Allergy Attack			
Recurring Skin Problem			

CONSENT FORM FOR MEDICAL TREATMENT

In the Event of a Medical Emergency Involving My Children Named

I Hereby Delegate _____ to Take Legal Responsibility for Decisions Concerning Their Medical Well-Being Should I Not Be Available to Give My Consent.
Signed _____Date _____
Relationship to the children_____

It is preferred that this form be notarized.

USING THE
TELEPHONE

COMMON
COMPLAINTS

MINOR
INFECTIONS

INFECTIOUS
DISEASES

EMERGENCY
PROBLEMS

NEW INFANT
CARE

PEDIATRIC
PROBLEMS

Index

USING THE TELEPHONE

COMMON COMPLAINTS

MINOR INFECTIONS

INFECTIOUS DISEASES

EMERGENCY PROBLEMS

NEW INFANT CARE

PEDIATRIC PROBLEMS

COMMON COMPLAINTS

MINOR INFECTIONS

INFECTIOUS DISEASES

EMERGENCY PROBLEMS

NEW INFANT CARE

PEDIATRIC PROBLEMS

USING THE TELEPHONE

COMMON COMPLAINTS

MINOR INFECTIONS

INFECTIOUS DISEASES

EMERGENCY PROBLEMS

NEW INFANT CARE

PEDIATRIC PROBLEMS

USING THE TELEPHONE

COMMON COMPLAINTS

MINOR INFECTIONS

INFECTIOUS DISEASES

EMERGENCY PROBLEMS

NEW INFANT CARE

PEDIATRIC PROBLEMS